Published by RiverRun Select
An imprint of Piscataqua Press and
RiverRun Bookstore
142 Fleet St | Portsmouth, NH 03801 | USA
603-431-2100 | www.riverrunbookstore.com

Printed in the United States of America

ISBN-13: 978-0-9856073-9-5

Library of Congress Control Number: 2012919987

www.piscataquapress.com

JUDY'S JOURNEY

By Earle Whitcher

This book is lovingly dedicated to the memory of

Judy L. Whitcher

My wife and best friend.

Foreword

Writers of fiction have the literary freedom to select a topic of choice, invent the meanderings through which the plot will flow, and finally, to determine the conclusion. Not so with non-fiction and biographical works. The course, the sequence, and the outcome have already been established and settled long before the words are committed to paper (or other forms of technology). The author's primary task in relaying a true story is to bring the details to life, conveying them to the reader in an honest and meaningful manner.

Judy's Journey is a true story. It is a lasting testament to a courageous woman, recounting the valiant battle she waged against breast cancer. It is detailed and descriptive, often in very colorful terms; it incorporates humor when appropriate; it is always respectful and considerate; but above all, it is genuine and honest in every aspect. Though a sobering chronicle, it is an inspiring account of one couple's determined struggle—together—against a fearsome opponent.

The development of a strong support network yielded multifaceted, invaluable benefits for the couple as they faced formidable circumstances. In retrospect, the author's use of computerized "updates" clearly demonstrated their value as an effective communication tool. Without doubt, they provided an emotional outlet as well. While never intended to draw attention to self, *Judy's Journey* also poignantly bears witness to the commitment made several decades earlier by Judy's

i

husband who promised to be by her side "in sickness and in health ... until death do us part."

I had the opportunity to re-read *Judy's Journey* numerous times before it was deemed ready for publication. Each time I reviewed the manuscript, I envisioned another potential target audience who could derive invaluable benefits from these experiences. Obviously, this would include those dealing with cancer or other life-threatening illnesses, as well as members of their families and friends. For cancer survivors, it is an affirmation of their personal struggles. It provides an adjunctive therapeutic intervention for those who have survived the loss of a loved one. It serves as a resource to individuals involved in healthcare, including educators and students in diverse associated fields. It contributes to better understanding and empathy for pastors, counselors, and for those whose ministry is that of encouragement and grief resolution. Finally, it is my personal opinion that *Judy's Journey* provides fertile ground for soul-searching for couples intending to enter into a committed marriage. It is a sobering reminder that no one can anticipate what the future may hold. It will enable them to seriously contemplate what the words of those vows—"in sickness and in health ... until death do us part"—really mean.

Judy's story, told from the powerful and intimate perspective of her husband, is an inspirational experience that deserves to be shared with others.

Anna M. Davis, Editor

Prologue

Although the majority of Judy's story takes place between May 2008 and February 2011, in reality, the account begins five years earlier, in 2003. In order to put all that I am about to relate in its proper perspective, some background would seem to be appropriate.

Early in 2003, while undergoing what had become a periodic routine eye exam to monitor the ongoing effects of glaucoma, Judy's ophthalmologist mentioned the disturbing, but not frightening—at least at the time—fact that he had identified something during the exam which he was not qualified to deal with. He set up an appointment for the next day with a noted local neurosurgeon. In hindsight, the fact that he had already arranged a "next day" appointment with a specialist to address this new discovery should have put us on immediate high alert. At the time however, we had no prior experience with neurosurgeons and had no idea that an appointment made that quickly signaled anything out of the ordinary. Our only thought was that perhaps this would explain the bothersome spots (referred to as floaters) which had recently started affecting Judy's vision.

Judy kept the appointment the next day, blissfully unaware of the potential impact of this event. She went alone, having declined both my offer and the offer of friends from work to accompany her to this fateful meeting. We had no way of foreseeing the significance of this appointment.

As Judy later recounted the story, "When the doctor's first words were, 'You have a brain tumor ... '" she admitted to having heard little else that he had to say. A state of shock, disbelief, and bewilderment overtook her entire being. This was far from the norm for someone who was normally poised, self-confident, and in control.

The subsequent treatment regimen required to deal with this unwelcome intruder was to dominate our lives for the next five years. Following surgical removal, it was determined that the tumor was benign, probably the product of some local brain cells that had simply gone into a reproductive frenzy. We were thankful that it was not the manifestation of a malignant cancer that had migrated from some other part of the body (referred to as a metastasis). The condition was nevertheless serious and posed significant danger. This was primarily due to the fact that the tumor had been wrapped around the optical nerve of the right eye, causing the nerve to be out of alignment. This was the reason for the troublesome spots in her visual fields. Had this tumor not been attended to, it could have led to more serious problems including blindness and possibly death from potential intracranial pressure. In spite of the seriousness and delicacy of the tumor excision due to its location, the neurosurgeon was confident that he could remove the offensive trespasser with no ill effects to Judy's well-being or personality.

The surgery was performed and, with the exception of a very strange haircut and the permanent loss of peripheral vision in her right eye, Judy survived the procedure, rebounding with her characteristically positive outlook. From that point on though, we lived in a state of ever-watchful apprehension and heightened anxiety as we continued the prerequisite follow-up tests right up to the final exam in April 2008. At that time, we reached the much-anticipated milestone of negative scans that signaled the "All Clear." We had achieved the goal for which everyone in similar situations strives. It had been five years with no indication of any recurrence of the tumor. After numerous MRI's, PET scans, and an array of other tests, the tumor was confirmed to be "history." The medical community standards declared that the condition had been cured.

I still remember that cool, spring day like it was yesterday. Following that momentous news, as we sat in the parking lot that day, we both breathed huge sighs of relief. It was as if an unbearable weight had been removed from our shoulders. Now after five long years, we thought we could get on with the rest of our lives. Little did we know what fate held in store for us.

In April 2008, at the time we were the recipients of this good news, I was 59, Judy was 57, and a month earlier we had celebrated our 39th wedding anniversary. Life was indeed good: we both had stable jobs which we liked; our family was comfortably grown, making their own ways in life; and we were blessed with the joy that is unknown until experienced—grandchildren.

This euphoria was to be short lived. The world was soon to come crashing down around us once again.

On May 4, 2008, Judy called me to her side, indicating a spot under her left arm that was strangely and alarmingly hard to the touch. Judy had always been mindful of her health. Even in our younger days when many of us took part in what we now recognize to have been risky practices, she was the steadfast and stalwart follower of the healthy and safer choices that so many of us spurned in the youthful denial of our mortality. She continued to adhere to these health-conscious routines throughout her adult life. She had followed all of the age-appropriate screening recommendations, tests, and procedures. In light of this, we were not overly concerned by the lump or the fact that her left breast was slightly engorged and had a pinkish tint; it appeared to be similar to a minor sunburn. Together, we decided that it would be best if she saw our doctor as soon as possible. The experiences of the past five years probably made us both more reactive than we might otherwise have been. Not one to procrastinate, she made and kept that appointment the next day.

The doctor's examination was inconclusive. He thought it might be a simple infection. In case this was the situation, he prescribed an antibiotic. He also wisely advised her to make an appointment at the local Women's Breast Health Center. That appointment, with professionals who deal with this type of condition on a daily basis, confirmed our worst fears. Judy was diagnosed with *Inflammatory Breast Cancer*, also known simply as IBC. As innocuous as it sounds, IBC is one of the rarest and most aggressive types of breast cancer. It affects about three to four percent of those stricken with breast cancer.

The initial shock and distress overwhelmed us. Once we recovered, we—and although I say we, I should say, Judy—determined to face this new challenge as she had everything in her life—head-on—with courage and the conviction that together we could deal with it, beat it, and move on.

On the day following the diagnosis, I asked Judy how she wanted to handle the situation. Did she want to circle the wagons and remain private and withdrawn, revealing information to only the closest of family members? Did she prefer to share the facts, as they became known, with any of our widespread family and friends who would want to know of her condition? In her usual pragmatic manner, she opted to be open and forthcoming. She determined that it would be better to be straightforward and honest with our supporters so that they would not have to endure months of misinformation, speculation, and innuendo.

What I hope to convey in this chronicle of our personal journey is the level of courage, dedication, and unwavering faith that Judy displayed in the face of overwhelming adversity. Most of us can only hope to aspire to these lofty goals should we find ourselves confronted with similarly harsh challenges in life. Judy maintained a level of hope, resilience, and determination that benefited her family and friends as much as it ministered to her. Indeed, although she often credited me with supporting her, it was in fact, she who sustained me and made it possible to "soldier" on through those most trying of times. She was an inspiration to all who were privileged to have known her. I will forever honor her memory and tell all who will listen about the bravest person I have ever known.

What follows is a compilation of emails that quickly became known simply as "updates." Some of my original messages have been altered slightly for several reasons: the removal of time constraints has permitted me to review grammar, punctuation, and syntax oversights—many of the updates were composed in haste and often during periods of extreme emotional stress; to provide additional explanations related to medical procedures and terminology for those unfamiliar with situations such as those we faced; and finally, for purposes of clarification, particularly for readers who have not had the benefit of "the rest of the story."

In assembling the updates into a cohesive format, I have also included commentaries which serve to introduce the circumstances surrounding the update which follows. These inserts chronicle some of the unspoken thoughts and emotions swirling around us. They also reveal more clearly now, in retrospect, some aspects which had been shrouded in a mist of confusion—and yes, sometimes even unconscious denial—as we lived the "journey."

It is important to note that our email support group was constantly adding newcomers who were eager for news regarding Judy's status. For the benefit of those who had recently joined us, there were several instances when I repeated previously shared information to which they may not have been privy earlier.

Though most of the original updates were generated by me, I discovered that there were additional personal messages through which Judy had also communicated with her family, friends, and co-workers. As I have reproduced Judy's communications, it has been my intent, as much as possible, to preserve the messages that she authored as she had written them.

I need to mention that although this collection may have been compiled by me, it was not my foresight that made this book possible. Its evolution was the result of a combination of factors: the incessant urging of one of Judy's cousins to attempt this undertaking; and the surprising discovery that a number of Judy's supporters, including her sister, had saved the entire collection of updates and so willingly forwarded them back to me when this project was still in its embryonic stage. It is to those friends and family and to Judy's memory that I must give credit for this volume. I can only hope that in some small way it will help others find the strength necessary to face their own trials with the courage and conviction that Judy displayed throughout her entire ordeal.

What you are about to read has been a difficult undertaking for me. First, because this type of endeavor is not something I have ever envisioned myself doing, and more significantly, because of the powerful emotional stirrings it has dredged up. The editing was so difficult that I had to perform the process in reverse; starting at the end and working backward to the beginning. Reliving those days was, at times, more than I ever thought I could bear. It required re-experiencing the highs and lows and knowing the content of the next chapter before getting there. In the end though, this has been a cathartic exercise for me. It has helped me to deal with unprecedented emotions as I forced myself to revisit what we all later recognized to be inevitable, but no one wanted to accept. I hope that my readers are able to draw a measure of strength and faith from my meager efforts. It is my desire that these words will offer encouragement to others in dealing with whatever crisis they, or their loved one, may face in their own lives.

I am hesitant to relate this because none of this was intended to be about me, but one of my "editors" insists that I include the fact that this account is also about honoring the vows I made to Judy before our family, friends, and God to "love and cherish" her "in sickness and in health ... until death do us part." While I do not purport to have done anything "above and beyond"—it was merely what I signed on for—if somehow it encourages another spouse to be there when needed for his or her mate, this journal will have served another serendipitous purpose.

To the many friends and family who followed our journey, I would be remiss if I did not take this opportunity to once again thank each of you for all of your support, prayers, and heartfelt wishes. It is not possible to overstate how much they meant to both of us during those overwhelming days as our lives unraveled. We drew strength and courage from the knowledge that so many dear friends and family were behind us and were upholding us at every turn. Thank you all for that generous and unselfish support.

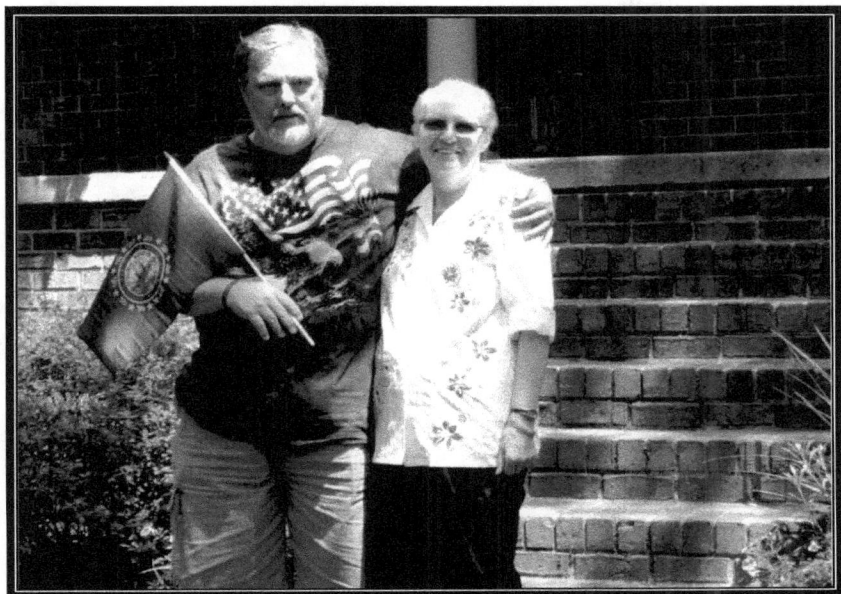

Judy & Earle

United we stand; together, in all things...

Introduction

What you are about to read is not an ordinary book in the conventional form of a novel. It is, nonetheless, a story—a very personal story of our family's torturous travels through the all too common experience of cancer diagnosis and treatment. Before beginning *Judy's Journey*, allow me to provide some background to better acquaint you with some of the characters whom you are about to accompany on this incredible journey.

Judy was born in a small town in Southern New Hampshire in July 1950. She was the second daughter of Pearl and Sylvia Davis. In addition to her parents, Judy's family consisted of an older sister and two younger brothers. She was a happy child and in her preteen years grew into something of a tomboy.

When she was about ten years old, her family moved approximately one mile from their former home. In doing so, they crossed a town line bringing Judy into my life for the first time; I was twelve. Her family moved two houses south of where my folks had settled just a year earlier. Over time, the two families went from being merely neighbors to friends; as a consequence, Judy and I saw each other often.

Judy's Journey

In the awkward teen years that soon followed, our relationship took a decided nosedive. For a few years, we were not even as much as on speaking terms. Throughout this time however, Judy became my mother's right hand. My father had passed away when I was fourteen. In addition to me, he left my mother a young widow with five active sons: aged from four years to just three months old. Judy was the one person upon whom she could always count when she needed help. This relationship continued to develop irrespective of the fact that Judy and I did not even acknowledge each other's existence. For both of us, it was an arrangement made easier by the fact that we went to different high schools and virtually never saw each other.

In the spring of 1967, I was a junior in high school and worked after school each day. My schedule was such that I came home rather late, especially on Friday nights when I worked a full 3-11 shift. One particular Friday, I came home to find the lights in the house were ablaze—a highly unusual situation. As an eighteen-year-old young man, my immediate thought was "What have I done that my mother has discovered?" It took an abnormally long time to park my car and enter the house that night. I was still not sure what was in store for me.

Upon entering, I found my mother sitting at the table with a cup of coffee; she was obviously waiting for me. "What could be the reason?" I wondered. She asked me to sit down and said "There's something that I want to talk to you about." I was certain that I was doomed. She proceeded to tell me of a sad turn of events that had befallen her close friend and trusted babysitter—actually, more like a nanny—Judy. Although Judy and I had not spoken or even seen each other for nearly three years at this point, I knew that she and my mother were close. Though I could understand her concern, I was at a loss to even begin to fathom how any of this could possibly involve me.

The situation was that Judy's Junior Prom was coming up soon—she would always correct me here when I told the story and remind me that it was not a Prom, but a Semi-Formal—I still don't know the difference. At any rate, Judy had been invited by a young man from her school. Understandably, she was looking forward to attending. Her folks had already bought a new dress for the occasion. The preparations were nearly complete when the young man backed out. To say that Judy was upset would be putting it mildly; devastated would be closer to the truth. However, she had come up with a backup plan, born of desperation, to help save face with her friends. She asked my mother, her friend and confidant, to speak to me about the possibility of being her escort to this major social event. To sweeten the bargain, if I would agree to do so, she would arrange a future date with one of her friends. I thought I knew the friend she would task with fulfilling this big favor so, after a little consideration, I agreed to the deal.

The big night came and we went to the dance in all of our 60's finery. The evening went well and I found myself actually enjoying the company of this charming young lady who had somehow taken the place of the tomboy I had known so long ago. I was not only

3

enjoying her company, I discovered that I was not tongue-tied and nervous as was normally the case with previous dating encounters. She was easy to talk to and pleasant to be with. I was enchanted with this demure young lady who, with her willowy figure and long, dark hair, reminded me of my then (still really) heart-throb, Cher. When the evening came to its inevitable end, I said to her "This has been fun. Would you like to do something again sometime?" Almost to my surprise, she agreed; and we were together from that point on. I should note here that I never did get that date with her friend and whenever I told this story, I always reminded her that she still owed me a date. She would just smile and shrug it off. If the truth be told, I have sometimes wondered if there ever was an intended date to be made or if Judy's plan had unfolded exactly as she intended.

We were married in the spring of 1969 and left rural New Hampshire to sample life on our own terms. We both agreed that anywhere had to have more to offer than the Granite State. I was serving in the U.S. Air Force at the time and our first duty assignment was Nellis AFB in Las Vegas, Nevada. It was reported in the local newspaper that we were "honeymooning in Las Vegas," but nothing could have been further from the truth. Vegas is not a fun place when you are an E-3 making poverty wages and underage to boot, thus unable to sample the excitement the town offered— even if we could have afforded it. We made the best of our time there though, and after nearly a year we left Nevada as a family of three. Our daughter, Christina joined us as we departed for our next adventure—

compliments of Uncle Sam—an assignment to Hahn Air Base in West Germany.

Through a series of unforeseen, cascading events, we spent four years in Germany. This was made possible by extending my enlistment after I made E-5 and qualified for an accompanied tour, provided that we served the full four year tour in Germany. While there, our family grew by one with the arrival of our son, Charles. We enjoyed our time in Europe and were fortunate to have experienced many things which would not have been possible otherwise. One of the most treasured benefits of our extended stay in Germany was the development of the lifelong friendships we came away with.

Early on, we befriended a group of young airmen who were stationed at Hahn following their training. Three of these airmen became members of my load crew when I was assigned as Crew Chief. There were several others who made up the larger group; most of them were single GIs. They all looked to Judy as their "Mother Hen." They would confide all sorts of things to her while seeking her advice, mostly on matters of the heart and regarding their girlfriends back home. We were a close group. Now, 40 years later, our friendships have continued to stand the test of time. We have been assembling for planned reunions for more than thirty years. These events continue to be more like family reunions than military gatherings. The "Hahn Family" as we came to think of this group was, and still is, an important part of our lives. These folks were a wellspring of love and support for both Judy and I throughout our ordeal.

5

In the years subsequent to the completion of my military service, we settled down near the area where we had grown up. We eventually built our home in the town of our youth; the same place from which we had declared our independence some ten years earlier. During this time, Judy became the consummate woman of the 20th century. In addition to being a mother and housewife (which included keeping me in line), she worked a full-time job to help with the household expenses. From the time it officially opened, Judy was employed as the shop clerk for the transportation department at the Wal-Mart Distribution Center nearby. As the only female employee in that department, she was often cast into the "Mother Hen" character for her Wal-Mart "Men" as she called them. It was quite similar to the role she had previously enjoyed with the single GIs at Hahn years earlier.

As time passed, our parents approached their twilight years. It was Judy's foresight that prompted us to set up revocable trusts for them as a way to ease the inevitable estate settlement intricacies which we fully expected would fall to us to resolve. Throughout their last years, Judy managed their medical and financial needs and arranged for homecare when it eventually became necessary. It was her honesty and sense of fairness, as well as her nurturing personality, that guided her to provide for the continued care of her siblings. These same qualities, coupled with Judy's genuine concern and willingness to extend herself for others, were endearing aspects that permeated Judy's entire life and made her such a dear friend to all who knew her.

Judy's philosophy of life was that "What will be, will be." She never expressed annoyance that "life wasn't fair" or indulged in "pity parties." She not only played the hand that she had been dealt, but did so in an admirable manner.

Now that you have become better acquainted with who we are, please join us as we relive those frightening, often joyous, yet always hopeful days that make up *Judy's Journey*.

Judy's Journey is based upon a collection of actual messages that became known as "updates" when they were sent out to family and friends whose initial numbers were approximately 30. Eventually, the recipients totaled in excess of 125 addressees. These missives follow the peaks and valleys of our personal journey. The communications provide the framework of this manuscript and underscore Judy's courage and strength as she engaged in her fight for survival in the face of the ominous curse of breast cancer.

From the onset, we both knew that the odds were heavily stacked against us as Judy was facing one of the most aggressive forms of breast cancer. Though known by the serene sounding name of *Inflammatory Breast Cancer*, it was anything but. The medical team was forthcoming with the treatment limitations. During treatment, we learned that the accepted protocol we were following had been approved a mere two years prior to Judy's diagnosis. The combination of chemotherapy, surgery, and radiation had proven effective in many cases, provided there was no metastasis.

When it was confirmed that the cancer had spread to the brain, we knew that the path we were traveling had changed irrevocably. We were now facing the inevitable. Our focus altered significantly as we accepted the fact that we were speeding toward a destination which we had hoped to avoid for several more years. Until the very end, we continued to hope against hope for a happier ending to Judy's story. However, it was not to be.

Though not intentional, this chronicle also serves to highlight the endurance of our marriage. It not only survived, but strengthened, throughout that battle. I consider our experience to be evidence of the indomitable human spirit that resides in all of us and comes to the forefront when called upon in such extraordinary circumstances as these.

This narrative is not a bid for your sympathy, but rather, it is my hope that it will inspire and encourage anyone who may find themselves—or their loved ones—in similar circumstances. It is intended as reassurance for all who may come this way; it is possible to live life to the fullest, regardless of what time limitations God may have set for that life.

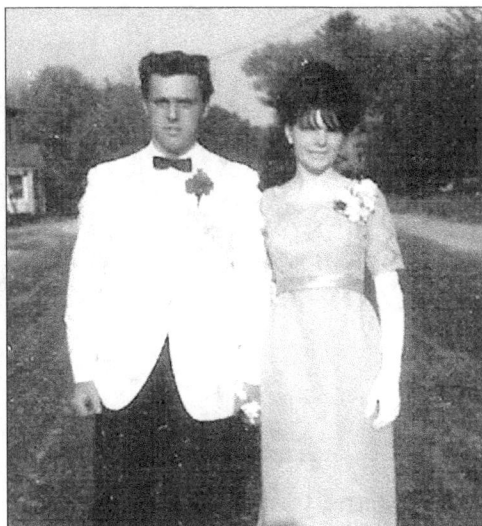

Earle and Judy all dressed up, departing on their first date

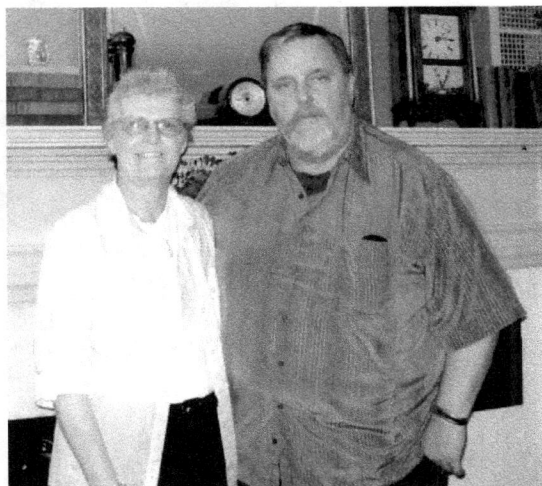

Judy and Earle celebrating their 40th Wedding Anniversary

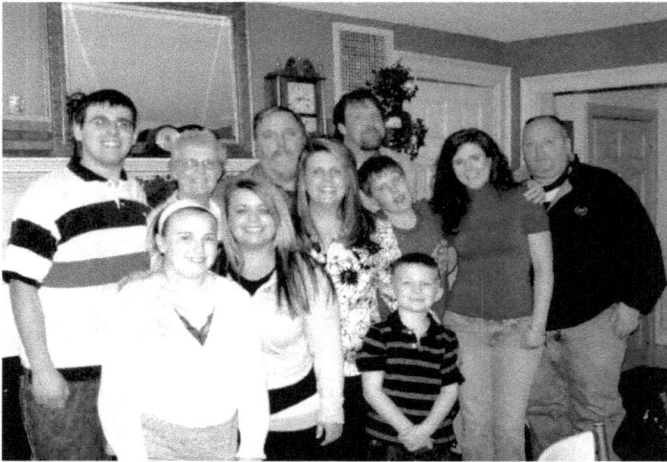

The entire family is gathered together to celebrate with them: Samantha, Cindy, Christina, Jeff Jr., Andrew, Julie, Jeff, Justin, Judy, Earle and Chuck

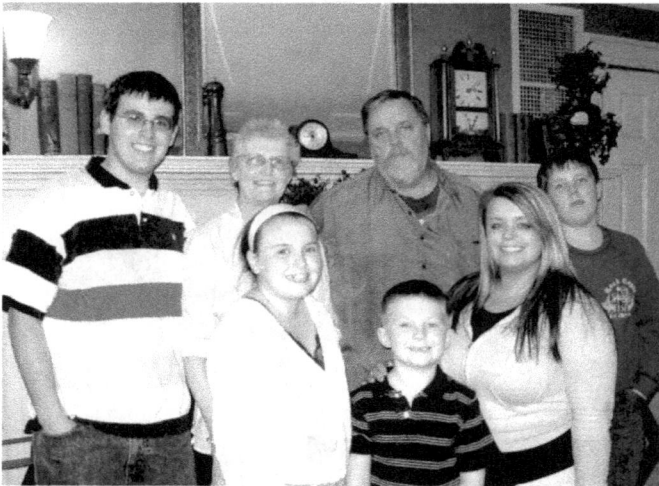

Judy and Earle with all five of their grandchildren: Justin, Samantha, Jeff Jr., Cindy, and Andrew

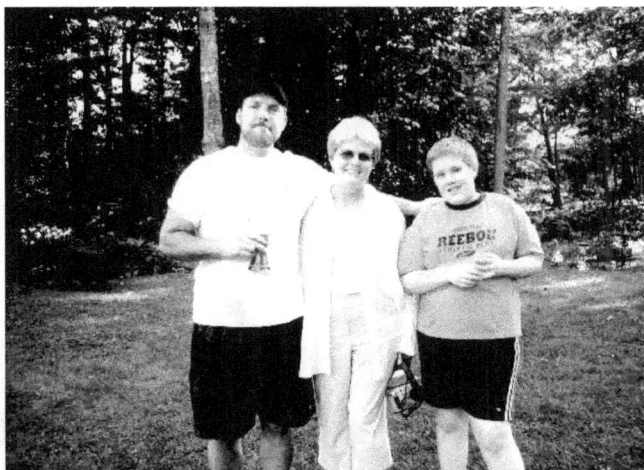

Judy with son Chuck and grandson Andrew

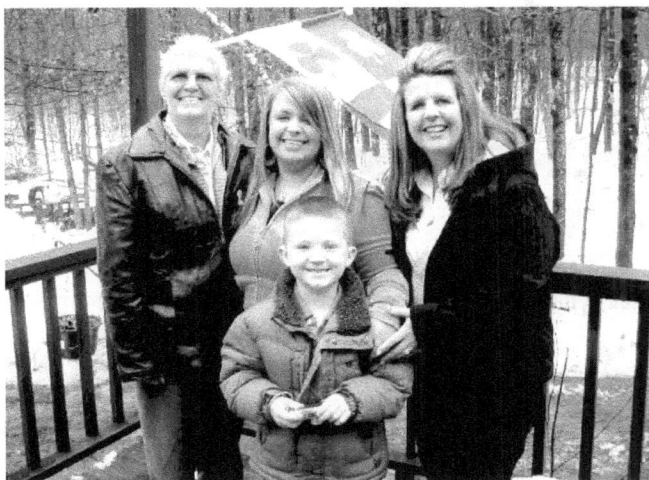

Judy with grandkids Cindy, Jeff Jr., and daughter, Christina

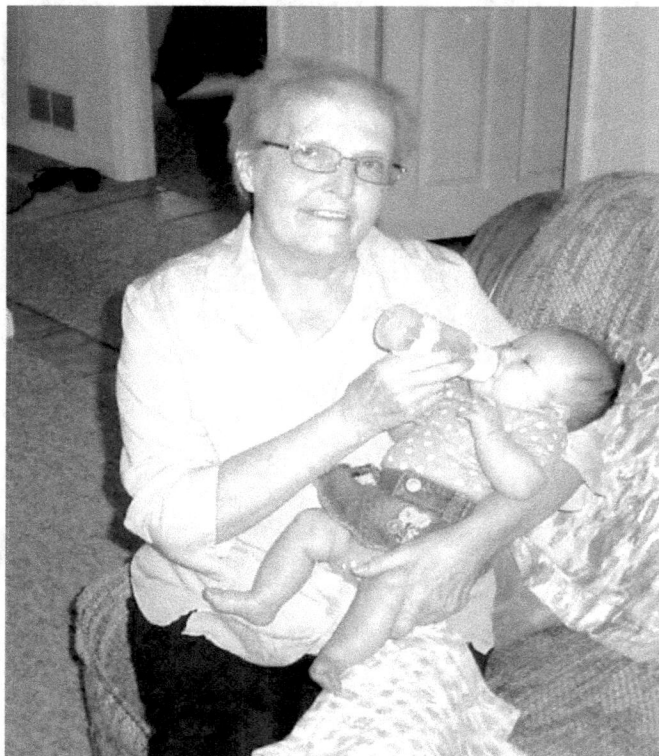

Judy, enjoying the new role of great-grandmother. Jaidyn was a special blessing for all of us at this difficult time.

2008

Judy's Journey

The Beginning

Judy's Journey begins in early May of 2008. Judy and I shared our hopes, our fears, our elations, and our disappointments with our many friends and family who hungered for news of Judy's condition. In return, they provided us with immeasurable support and encouragement, as well as prayer sustenance, and reaffirmations of faith that bolstered our commitment to each other to carry on in the greatest battle of our lives. What follows are the messages, or "updates" as they became known. They carried the news of the ongoing confrontation as it unfolded. Judy's story is one of strength, determination, and perseverance in the face of a deadly adversary. It's not so much about how the battle culminates; it's about purposeful tenacity; it's about the valiant fight waged with the weapons modern medicine can so effectively launch; and finally, it's about the dedication of the healthcare team who made it all happen. *Judy's Journey* is a testament to Judy's courage and resolve. May it be an inspiration to all those who follow her journey.

Judy's Journey

Tuesday, May 6, 2008

Dear Friends & Family,

This note is to inform you—not alarm you—so read all the way through before jumping to any conclusions.

Sunday, Judy brought to my attention the fact that she had found a rather large lump under her left arm. There was some swelling, discoloration, and discomfort in the surrounding areas as well. She was scheduled for a mammogram the following Tuesday, but we agreed that she should call our doctor the next day, Monday. She did so and was seen right away.

The P.A. *(physician's assistant)* and the doctor both examined her and then sent her for blood work and a sonogram. The blood work came back and was encouraging. The sonogram showed a large, deeply embedded tumor in the lymph nodes. In addition to these tests, she was sent to the Breast Cancer Center for another exam and to try to draw some fluid from the tumor. They did not aspirate any fluid, but did get enough material to send out for a biopsy. The results of that are expected tomorrow, Wednesday. In the interim, she is taking an antibiotic in an effort to reduce the swelling and inflammation.

We won't know what the next step will be until some results come in, but it seems reasonable to expect an MRI to get a full picture of what is going on. There is a strong possibility that surgery may be needed in the future as well, but we cannot be sure of that until we know more. At this point, there is no reason to think this

16

is anything more that an unwanted, unwelcome lump. We are following the doctor's advice and we are highly optimistic that this will become just a footnote in Judy's medical history when it is all over. We will keep you updated as more information becomes available.

Earle & Judy

> At this juncture, we were holding our collective breaths hoping for a favorable report from the initial tests. Judy had experienced lumps in the past. In the previous situations, medical evaluations always determined them to be calcium deposits. We were praying that this would turn out to simply be another of those.

Wednesday, May 7, 2008

Today came and went with mixed news. On the positive side, the antibiotics seem to be helping. Some of the swelling is going down. Also, two more results from the blood tests came in. Both brought good news. One thing that we were expecting did not come in: the biopsy results. As all the other reports are in a positive vein, we are not overly concerned about the lack of news from the biopsy. In the end though, the biopsy results are key to deciding what type of action we will need to follow. Overall, we are encouraged by the news we have thus far, but we are still delaying any celebration until we get the biopsy results.

Judy's Journey

We take this opportunity to thank you all for your encouraging words and for keeping us in your prayers.

We will send more news when it becomes available.

Earle & Judy

We still do not have the definitive report from the biopsy and are continuing in a holding pattern. All reports that we have received to date have been good news so we are cautiously optimistic at this point. The doctor's office will not provide any information over the phone, but they have scheduled an appointment.

Thursday, May 8, 2008

Not much to report today. The doctor's office called and set up an appointment for tomorrow morning to discuss the biopsy results with Judy. We should have a better handle on what they have found and what course of action to expect. I'll pass this along when we know more.

Thank you for all your prayers and encouragement.

Earle & Judy

The day of truth has arrived. We approached this appointment with a great deal of trepidation and apprehension. We are still hopeful and outwardly upbeat.

Friday, May 9, 2008

(*Big Breath*)   The news is in—and it is not as we had hoped.   The ominous diagnosis has been confirmed. Judy has Inflammatory Breast Cancer.

A detailed explanation is available if you access the link below:

(The previous link has been omitted as it no longer appears to be active.)

It is too much to go into here, but suffice it say, it is rare, aggressive, and very serious.   The doctors are on top of the situation and we expect Judy will be scheduled for an MRI next week.   We also expect that she will be starting a course of treatment that will probably include chemotherapy, surgery, and radiation.

The road ahead looks as though it will be long and rough, but we will face it together and get past this.

Thanks to all for all your good thoughts and prayers.

Earle & Judy

> This was the first personal note I discovered from Judy to her friends and co-workers.   This was not one of the quasi-official updates.   It was strictly a personal message, but it provides insight into Judy's reaction to the news that we had just received.

Judy's Journey

Sunday, May 11, 2008

I didn't think I had so many tears inside of me, I think I could fill a lake.

http://www.ibcresearch.org/

Nothing new to report, but a close friend sent me this link and after checking it out, it seems to be a very good source of information. I especially like that it is written more for the layman to understand, [rather] than someone with a medical background. I found some of the links within the site very helpful and informative.

Judy

> Now we begin what was to become the first of many false starts and disappointing delays—all in the name of safety for Judy, but nonetheless, discouraging and disheartening for both of us.

Thursday, May 15, 2008

It is difficult to know where to even start this update. Judy had her MRI today and we had expected to have some more definitive information following the procedure. Instead, we are less sure of what is going on than before.

The MRI showed two small tumors in the affected breast, but the doctor said they were so small that they couldn't be the cause of what is happening. They discovered that the lymph nodes are plugged and loaded with cancer. They also found that there is an unidentified spot on her liver. This may turn out to be nothing more than a cyst, but until we know for certain what it is, we cannot proceed.

The medical team has determined that she is in Stage III. If the spot on the liver turns out to be malignant, then she would be considered at Stage IV. At this point, the course of treatment we will be following will depend on the outcome of tests concerning the liver.

We will see the oncologist Monday afternoon when they will do a PET scan. Following that, we will sit down with him to discuss what course of action we will be pursuing. We expect to have more information subsequent to that appointment.

In the meantime, thank you for all your positive thoughts and prayers.

Earle & Judy

> Now we introduce the phrase we will use all too often in this and future updates: "we have a mixed bag to report." Though the news could not be termed bad, it was still not all that we had hoped to hear.

Monday, May 19, 2008

We have had our initial meeting with the oncologist and there is a mixed bag to report. First, the best news: there was no indication of any problem with the suspicious spot on the liver. The news we did expect, however, was confirmed. The original diagnosis stands: Judy does have Inflammatory Breast Cancer. I'll include the link that explains about this disorder in case I missed anyone earlier.

The next step is not a PET scan, but a CT scan and some kind of test to establish a baseline heart function because one of the chemotherapy drugs she will be receiving occasionally affects the heart. With a baseline, they will have something to compare to throughout the process. We will meet the nurses on the 31st to learn what to expect during the treatments.

Treatments are scheduled to start June 2nd. The overall plan is as we expected: chemotherapy, surgery, radiation, and possibly additional chemo. The doctor seemed quite confident that even though this is one of the more aggressive cancers, with an equally aggressive treatment plan we can beat it. That was more than a little comforting to hear.

Thanks to all for your good thoughts and for keeping us in your prayers.

Earle & Judy

The process is moving forward at its own pace. Here, I remind the recipients—as I will do often in the future—not to despair when there is a gap in the updates. Everyone seems to be so anxious for news that I must plead with all to remember that "no news is good news." It was a concept they found difficult to embrace.   Judy and I soon realized that we had seriously underestimated the urgent desire that the recipients would demonstrate for the latest news on Judy's condition.

Friday, May 30, 2008

In case you were wondering what happened to the updates, rest assured that in this case "no news is good news." There has been very little to report as the week has been spent undergoing tests and checking out wigs. I asked Judy to consider a wig with red hair. She was less than receptive to the suggestion. I thought it was a perfect opportunity to be married to a redhead for a while. (At some point in the future, Judy would compromise with a lightly tinted auburn wig.)

All the tests have been completed now.   Early this morning, she had a port installed. *(A port is a medical reservoir that is implanted just beneath the skin surface to "receive" injectable medications.   It eliminates the need for repeated skin punctures when IVs and other injections are required.)* This afternoon, we went to the treatment center for our orientation.   There was a LOT of information to take in, but I think we'll get it all under control.   Her treatments will take about three hours, with the first hour dedicated to pretreatment tests, blood work, red and white cell counts, and the like. Once these assessments have been completed and results have been confirmed to meet the prescribed criteria, she goes out back to the treatment room where she   will   get   the   actual   chemotherapy   drug administration.

The chemo administration process is expected to take about two hours. Once completed, it's back home with a strict directive: FOLLOW THE INSTRUCTIONS.

She will be going in for four treatments, one every other week. It takes that long for the blood counts to bounce back to the required levels in order to be able to withstand another round.

This is the first portion of the total program. She starts her first infusion on Monday, June 2nd. I will be taking her for this first round so that I can get a handle on the procedure. I may be recruiting some of the people who have already volunteered to help with transportation as the process moves forward, but we are all set for now.

Thanks to all for your kind words and prayers. We sincerely appreciate them.

Earle & Judy

At this point in the treatment process, I was still working full-time and could foresee logistical hurdles in the future. Fortunately, many of our supporters were in a position to offer more than emotional support and volunteered to help with transportation. They provided other additional much appreciated assistance as well.

Just as we were becoming adjusted to what was now our reality, the next devastating revelation from the doctors was delivered.

Monday, June 2, 2008

I have been pondering what to say and how to say it since we learned of the latest developments. If you will bear with me a moment and let me get my baseball metaphors in order, I'll bring you all up to date on the situation.

Last week was a busy time for Judy. She went through all sorts of tests, scans, and appointments. Today was to be our day to "Step up to the plate." We were prepared to do this. We were prepared for the "Fast Ball." We expected the "Fast Ball." We braced ourselves for the "Fast Ball" and they threw us a "Curve Ball."

It seems the CT scan showed that the cancer had possibly spread to some additional lymph nodes in the chest. Before we will be able to continue with the planned treatment, we will have to resolve the question concerning whether or not the lymph nodes are, in fact, cancerous or merely responding to an infection. To determine this, Judy will have a biopsy of the affected nodes and then possibly a PET scan.

At this time, we are expecting to resume the planned treatment program with the first treatment now rescheduled for the 16th of June. This has been a disturbing and disappointing development, but we continue to pursue a positive approach and move ahead per the doctor's protocols. The steps he is recommending are prudent and appropriate considering these new discoveries. We will keep you updated as this continues to unfold.

Thank you for your kind thoughts and prayers.

Earle & Judy

> The tempo of the progression is picking up. There is a sense of urgency even among the medical staff. This increased pace is still not fast enough for me as evidenced in this short note.

Tuesday, June 3, 2008

This will be a quick update as things are happening fast. First, the PET scan has been approved. Judy will undergo it tomorrow morning. This is good. The PET scan is the most complete test available to identify what the doctor needs to know in order for him to proceed effectively.

On Thursday, Judy will have a consultation with the doctor who will later be performing the biopsy. We have been told that the biopsy could take place as early as Friday. The sooner the better as far as I'm concerned. Once the results are known, we will find out when the treatment schedule will start. We will keep you updated as things happen.

Thank you for all your thoughts and prayers, they do help.

Earle & Judy

Friday, June 6, 2008

First and foremost, let me put everyone's mind at ease. Many have been anxious because there has been no update for a couple of days. When there is no news, there will be no update. I will only send these out when there is news. As I said before, this is a perfect example of "no news is good news."

Now, for today's surprising and upbeat update: today was a busy day. Judy was scheduled for her surgical biopsy this afternoon. We got a call this morning setting everything back an hour due to a change in the doctor's schedule. That was OK as it gave us a little extra time to do some other things before heading to the hospital.

We went in for the 2:00 p.m. registration and what we thought was to be the 3:00 p.m. procedure. Surprise, the procedure was at 4:00 p.m. Oh well, no problem.

While we were waiting, we discussed where we would stop for dinner on the way home. Then the doctor stopped by just before Judy went into the OR and informed us that she would be staying overnight for observation. We were "AH, AH, AHH. OK." You know what they say about "the best laid plans of mice and men ..."

The nice thing about having a plan is that you always know from where to deviate when something like this happens. That concludes the surprise part. Now, for the good news! The doctor was able to get to the nodes that were suspect from the CT scan and determined that they were all non-malignant! This was the best possible outcome for which we could have hoped. This means we are back to our original plan. We expect to be on track as of the 16th when Judy is scheduled for the first chemo treatment.

When I left the hospital, Judy was out of the recovery stage and in a room. I stayed until she was able to get some food. Remember, for this procedure she had to fast since 9:00 the night before; now it is 7:00 p.m. the next day.

At my departure, she was still in some pain from the surgery, but doing OK. She was watching the ball game and had devoured her supper. She is expected to come home tomorrow morning. I'll send along a new update on her condition when she gets home.

Thanks again for all your kind thoughts and prayers. We are certain they all help.

Earle & Judy

The next entry is Judy's personal message to her friends and family members letting them know she is home.

At this point, my updates are absent for a short time due to the fact that my laptop had to go into the shop. My updates resumed on June 16, some nine days later.

Saturday, June 7, 2008

I am home and resting. My nurses all told me I was a very sweet lady and a wonderful patient. That's because I always cleaned my plate when they brought me something to eat. HA. HA. I did well, took NO pain medicine and just did everything I was told to do. I know that is a surprise to some of you.

Thanks for all the prayers and good wishes you sent to me.

Judy

> The next two entries are again personal messages from Judy. In the first communication, she mentions the container of inspirational messages that her work family had presented to her. She saved all of the notes of encouragement in a lovely vase etched with flowers. Judy would often draw from the well of spirit-bracing messages when she needed a lift.
>
> In her next email she recounts a night out with friends two days later. The night out was a tremendous boost to her spirits at a time when delays and unexpected discoveries were working to dampen her normally positive, optimistic outlook.

Thursday, June 12, 2008

I wanted to share a very touching moment that happened to me today. The Wal-Mart Transportation

Judy's Journey

Team gave me a very special and precious gift today. They designed a beautiful glass vase filled with inspirational messages and favorite sayings. Each one is wrapped in a ribbon. I will start opening one a day when my treatments start on Monday.

The messages came from all my friends in the Bentonville, Arkansas office and my support group in Raymond, NH. There are 365 ribbon-wrapped messages. I can't tell [you] how much that touched my heart and Earle's.

My Wal-Mart family members are way too good to me, but I love it and soak up every precious minute they give me. I am so lucky to work with such a wonderful group of people and a great caring company. They are way too good to me; I don't deserve all the special attention they give me. I do keep them smiling with all my new hairdos which I'll be sharing with everyone as soon as I get a chance to take some pictures.

Judy

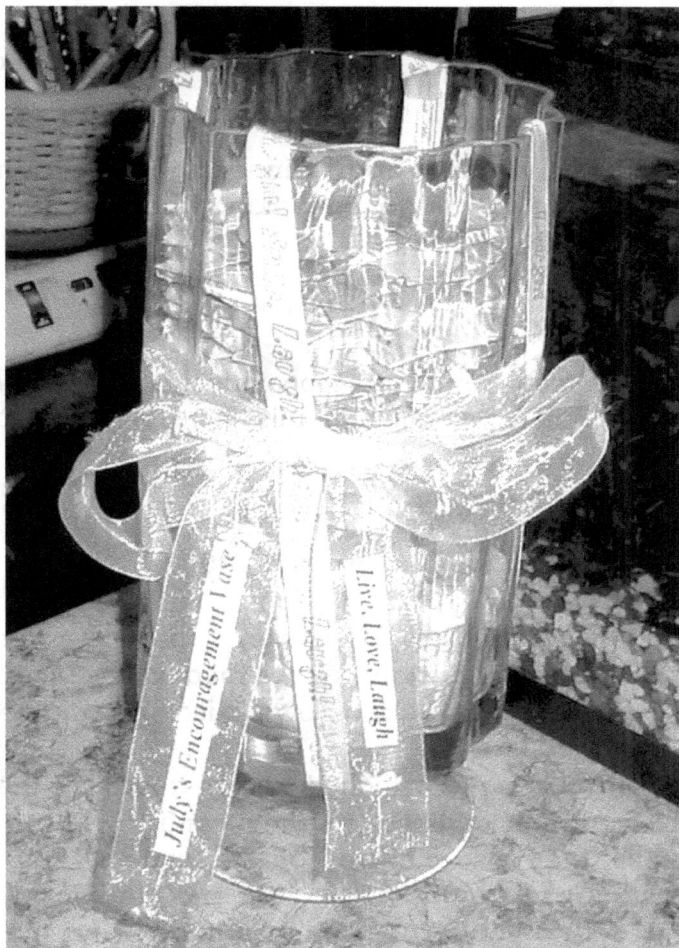

Judy's inspirational support vase contained uplifting and
encouraging messages.

Saturday, June 14, 2008

We went out to supper tonight with some friends. They wanted to treat me to a support dinner. We had a great time.

As I said, this was a support dinner so I'm all pumped up because they all said I am looking good.

Judy

> Next, we relate another disappointment. These would become all too familiar in this increasingly tedious process.

Monday, June 16, 2008

We have returned from the doctor and once again, we have to report the good news/bad news scenario. Actually, it's more like good news/ discouraging news.

First, the good news which is really good: all the test results are back and though they confirm the original diagnosis, they also clear all of the suspect sites. The lymph nodes in the chest are clear and the spots on the liver are of no concern. This was huge—and the best news we could have hoped for.

The downside is that the incision from the chest biopsy has not healed sufficiently to allow us to start chemotherapy. Due to the increased risk of infection, we have decided to wait another week to see if the healing progresses enough to reduce the additional risk of infection. We agreed that it is best to take the safer route and get the wound healed before we start the treatments.

So once again, we are in the starting blocks and the start has been delayed. As discouraging as this is, we feel confident that we are making the right decision. In the interim, Judy has been experiencing increasing signs and symptoms, but is holding up well. We are anxious to get underway and look forward to having better news to report next week.

Thanks to all for your thoughts and prayers, we are certain they help.

Earle & Judy

Finally, the news we have been anxiously waiting to report: the treatments have started. It has been approximately a month and a half since the original diagnosis was made and we are relieved to finally be underway. *Judy's Journey* has begun in earnest.

Monday, June 23, 2008

Here it is: news as it happens. Seriously, we just returned from the third try and as the old saying goes, "The third time is the charm."

The process was successful. We have finally started the chemo. The first session took four hours including all the lab prerequisites and the paperwork. The next session should be a little quicker. The port worked perfectly and made the process much easier. Judy did get sleepy when one of the drugs was started, but that was after she managed to beat me soundly in a game of cribbage.

She has to return tomorrow for a shot that helps boost her white cells. They want to see her on the Mondays between treatments to evaluate how well she is tolerating the meds. The final word is that the treatments have been started and we are confident that they will be successful.

The treatment center and the staff are both exceptional. They are accommodating, cordial, and thorough as well as highly professional. We are both glad that Judy is in their care.

Nothing else to report; just that the has started and we are thankful that you are keeping us in your thoughts and prayers.

Earle & Judy

This is another short note from Judy to her friends relating her current condition and how she is feeling. This was written on a Friday at the end of the work week and is an insight into what a toll the treatments are taking on her.

Friday, June 27, 2008

Today is a good day. I put in six hours at work and probably could have done seven, but didn't. I'm getting ready to take my nap.

My stomach felt good today. I didn't have to take any meds at all. I feel good right now and I'm ready for my afternoon nap, like I promised Earle.

I just wanted to share with you that today has been the best day of the week so far.

Judy

Monday, June 30, 2008

Today, Judy had her follow-up to check on how well she is tolerating the treatment and to assess how she is doing in general. In a nutshell, she passed with flying colors.

Her white count is where they expected it to be. That means she is rebounding from the initial chemo and that her dietary regimen is on track, accomplishing what is necessary in order for her body to be sufficiently recovered to withstand the next round. She received a positive review on all aspects that the "medical types" monitor.

It was an encouraging visit and we are both greatly pleased with the progress to date.

Judy's Journey

Thanks to everyone for your continued thoughts and prayers. We are certain that they all help.

Earle & Judy

The pace is picking up now. It has only been one week since the follow-up and a mere two weeks since the first chemotherapy treatment. We are pleased to finally be underway in the treatment program, but are still a little overwhelmed at the intricacy of the process.

Monday, July 7, 2008

Judy's second round of chemo was today. There is quite a process to get through before they actually administer the chemo drug. They do blood work to ascertain that her white count is at a level that will support the treatment.

During the interim, between treatments Judy is following a dietary regimen that is designed to boost her white count. Following the first chemo, her white count dropped from 7.3 to 2.6. However by following all of the instructions to the letter, she brought her count up to 9.1. This was good. It shows that she is able to rebound between chemo treatments and is better able to withstand the next round.

The doctor also noted that the drugs were already showing signs they were affecting the cancer. The pink tint is not as noticeable. The affected breast is not as heavy (due to relieving the blockage in the lymph nodes) and the lymph nodes themselves are not as hard.

Our son Chuck took Judy to this round of chemo and apparently they made quite the social day of it. One of the front desk receptionists had been his Sunday school teacher in the past. Also, while waiting with Judy in the treatment room, he encountered the parents of one of his classmates from 15 years ago.

So far, it appears that Judy has withstood the second round as well as can be expected. The anti-nausea meds seem to be working. She was able eat and keep down a small plate of food at supper time. She is very tired, but this seems to be a normal side effect of the chemo. Maybe it is the body's way of saying: "Time to rest."

All is well from here. We are greatly encouraged by the progress Judy is making.

Again, thanks to everyone for their prayers and good thoughts. There is no doubt that they all help.

Earle & Judy

This is a personal message from Judy to her boss at work. They had a close working relationship and often communicated with each other on matters of treatment and progress.

In this message, Judy again mentions her support jar. This was a large, glass, vase-shaped container that her co-workers had filled with inspirational messages similar to fortune cookie messages. She often pulled notes from this resource when she was in need an emotional boost. She drew much comfort from these snippets of encouragement.

Wednesday, July 9, 2008

The 3rd day after my chemo seems to be my hardest day. I did make it to work today, but only got 5 ½ hours in. I came home, had a cup of soup, took a nap, and watched my Red Sox Game.

I have pulled another message from my support jar and want to share it with you. *"In this life we get only things for which we are willing to sacrifice"*. Thank you whoever submitted that to my jar. You have brightened my day.

Thanks,

Judy

At the time of this message, we are two treatments into the program. We have embarked upon the roller coaster ride which will become all too familiar in the days, weeks, and months ahead.

Monday, July 14, 2008

This is the week for the "between treatments" evaluation. In general, the checkup went well, but there were some differences since the last medical exam. It turns out that Judy's red cell count was down. Although not at a dangerous level, it was at a point that required attention. This is a common situation for those receiving chemo, so it did not take the staff by surprise.

To combat the anemia, the decision was made to give her a shot of Procrit. This is a drug which stimulates the production of red cells. This should provide some relief from the increasing fatigue that she has been experiencing since the last chemo treatment. She has a long list of "Dos and Don'ts" as well as some changes in diet while adhering to this program. We are still adjusting to the new scheme of things, but Judy reports that she already feels more energy than she had in the previous few days.

Thanks to all for your continued thoughts and prayers, we do appreciate them.

Earle & Judy

We are at the point of the third chemotherapy treatment now. We believe that we are finally becoming accustomed to the system and how the process works. There is some good news this time. We are both pleased and thankful to be able to share it.

Judy's Journey

Monday, July 21, 2008

Today was Judy's third session of chemo. The lab work (blood testing), which is the initial phase of each session, went well. The injection that she received last week to boost her cell count did its work and she was cleared for the session. Except for some delay in getting started, the treatment went well.

The extra time that it took to get underway threw Judy's schedule off. She returned home very tired. She is resting now, but I fully expect her to bounce back.

The doctor has also ordered a cardiac evaluation. This is required at this point because some of the chemotherapy drugs that she is receiving can adversely affect the heart. It is intended to assess how well everything is being tolerated by her system.

The doctor's exam, performed prior to the chemo administration, went better than expected. He was unable to locate the nodule in the lymph node that had been quite noticeable just two weeks earlier. This is great news; it is an indication that the chemo is working. We are all encouraged by this latest development, since it indicates some very positive results.

Judy's spirits remain high. She is still putting in five to six hours per day at work. We laugh and joke about whatever we can, whenever we can. The fact that she is staying active pleases the doctor. He says that is a good sign.

As always, we are grateful for your thoughts and prayers. You are all in our hearts. We are certain this is helping. Thanks again.

Earle & Judy

Here is another of Judy's personal notes in which she shares some of her observations with her friends and co-workers. The subject of the support container comes up again. I didn't know at the time how much comfort she derived from this special gift from her friends at work. It is quite obvious that it meant a great deal to her.

Though Judy was still officially working at this point, the effort it took to get up and go into the Distribution Center was starting to challenge her remaining strength. Shorter days, and occasional days off, were becoming more frequent and a necessity. I was still working full-time at this juncture. Unfortunately, my schedule left Judy alone to deal with her emotions during the day.

Thursday, July 24, 2008

[I] wanted to let you know that it has been a tough couple of days for me. I have been home because we had a lot of guests at our shop this week and my boss and I decided it would be best for me to take a couple of days off.

Well, he made a very wise decision for me, because this round of chemo has knocked me off my feet. I have

41

no [sense of] taste so I don't want to eat. I have no desire to drink anything but [know that] I have to and it turns my stomach. [My sense of] smell has finally started to bother me so I really don't even want to make Earle supper or anything. I have pulled another slip from my support jar: *"Life is too short for a bad day!"* This is so true ...

I'm going to try and go into work tomorrow, just to see if it will take my mind off my discomfort. I'm doing my best to eat and drink to keep [myself] out of the hospital. [I] don't want to end up there.

We have made it through this terrible storm we had here today. Chris is OK. We are still trying to find out if Chuck's house is OK. His roads are closed and we are not sure if he can even get home. We are still waiting for him to call us.

Love,

Judy

It has been almost three months to the day since the initial diagnosis; the first full round of chemo has now been completed. This was an important milestone. Judy remains positive and upbeat in spite of the physically draining effects the treatments continue to have on her.

The reference in the following message was related to the confidence we had in the medical staff and doctors managing her treatment program. It was intended to assuage the occasional comment that we heard from some friends and family members wondering why we did not opt for treatment in Boston. We truly had the utmost trust in our team of healthcare providers. We also knew that they had access to the Boston expertise should it be needed. Finally, and most importantly, Judy was adamant that she would fight this with everything within her, but only with "accepted treatment protocols." She expressly communicated her reluctance to become involved in any experimental procedures.

Saturday, August 5, 2008

Well, a milestone of sorts has been reached. Judy has been for her fourth and final chemo in the initial stage of the treatment program. This concludes the first stage, but not the treatments. She has come through a little more tired than following the previous sessions, but as we were told, that was to be expected. Because the rounds of chemotherapy are cumulative, the after effects are likely to increase in intensity as the treatments proceed.

She managed to get a good night's sleep (very important) and is feeling up to tackling today. This afternoon, she gets the booster shot that typically knocks her feet out from under her.

The doctor was pleased with the continued progress of the treatments and was not able to digitally locate any lumps. This does not mean the cancer is gone, but it does mean that it is responding to the treatments. This is good.

Judy's Journey

On August 18th, Judy is slated to start the next round of chemo. This will involve a different set of chemicals with different procedures and, in all probability, different side effects as well. We are confident that Judy is up to this. Her spirits are high and we have full confidence in the doctor and the medical staff that we are dealing with.

Thanks to all for your continued support, prayers, and thoughts. We are certain they help.

Earle & Judy

> Now we start the second round of chemo. We learn exactly what the differences are—and that they are formidable. The meds are stronger and their effect is proportional to the increase in potency. This is also the first time we are introduced to the preventive compound called Herceptin. It was to play a major role in Judy's treatment in the forthcoming months.

Monday, August 18, 2008

Today was the first treatment of the second round of chemo. It was a very <u>LONG</u> day. The appointment was for 8:30 a.m. We finally left the center at 3:30 p.m. This was a double treatment with both the Taxol and the Herceptin. (I know, I know—I had to copy the names from the informational papers they gave us, otherwise I wouldn't have been able to come close to repeating them or have a clue on how to spell them.) The Taxol apparently is the heavy duty poison that takes almost four hours to administer. The Herceptin isn't as harsh; its "delivery" was completed in a little over an hour.

Judy slept through most of the administration of the heavy duty stuff and was just waking up when I returned from my assigned errands. After all, she wouldn't want me to have too much idle time on my hands. All kidding aside, besides being an efficient use of time, it kept me occupied.

The immediate results seem not to be as bad as the first treatment. She is awake, alert, and active. We'll see how things progress as time goes on.

She will be getting the treatments every week for eight weeks, but the double-dose administrations are scheduled for every other week. At the alternate week visit, she will only get the Herceptin which should be easier to tolerate.

The exam before the treatment was quite encouraging. The doctor was not able to detect the tumor at all. In fact, he referred to his notes a couple of times, then rechecked Judy, and declared that he was "very pleased with the way the treatments are going to date." He indicated that "there is every reason to think that we are on track to beat this."

This was the best news we could have received and we are equally encouraged.

Earle & Judy

Judy's Journey

This is another of Judy's personal notes. This one is addressed to her supervisor at work. Everyone she worked with has been concerned and actively following her progress. Additionally, many of her co-workers provided transportation and companionship when Judy was housebound.

The support jar is mentioned again, but something else must be noted as well. It is the first indication that Judy is concerned about the progress of the treatments and her ability to withstand them.

Wednesday, August 20, 2008

I call this "Awful Wednesday." It just seems I can't have a good Wednesday after treatment. I only worked four hours today [and] barely made that. [I] came home, got into my warm PJ's and went to bed. Slept about five hours and now [my] body really hurts—back, fingers, neck—but it's OK.

I pulled a support slip from my jar and here's what it reads: *"When nothing goes right, keep doing right"*!!! Guess I will have to just keep doing what I'm doing, knowing it will get better.

My biggest worry is [that] I don't have two weeks to get ready for a treatment now because they are every Monday. Sure hope this body is ready to tackle this. Thank you to whoever put that saying in the jar. We will see what tomorrow will hold.

Love,

Judy

The roller coaster ride that held us captive continues. An unexpected problem is discovered during the pretreatment checkup. We are about to encounter another disappointing delay, not to mention additional appointments with the eye doctor.

Judy continues to hold up well to these dilemmas as they crop up. In fact, because she was so unperturbed by these disruptions, it enabled me to deal with them much better than I would have otherwise. I could only guess at what she felt inwardly; outwardly she was a pillar of strength.

Monday, August 25, 2008

Today's report brings somewhat disappointing news— not devastating, but it is nonetheless, disheartening.

When Judy went for her treatment today, they discovered that her white count was extremely high. In fact, it was 43; high single numbers are desirable (7-9). They were initially concerned that this might be due to an infection, but that turned out not to be the case.

Apparently, the booster shot and the first round of the new chemo inadvertently interacted to really wring out her white cell production. Though this was a concern, the pivotal problem manifested itself when she revealed to the doctor that her vision was blurry.

After a round of pointed questions and consultations, her oncologist decided that she should see her ophthalmologist immediately. (*In the world of medicine,*

47

"immediately" is usually referred to as STAT and it means "now.") Before long, we would get to know that "now" meant right now, not next week, not even tomorrow. As we traveled this unfamiliar road, we would experience numerous occasions when we would leave one specialist to immediately be seen by another, often with no scheduled appointment.

Judy's eye doctor's office was contacted, the situation explained, and an immediate appointment was made for her. After the examination, it was determined that her near-sighted values had been affected. She has another appointment with the ophthalmologist on Sept. 5th. He will make recommendations at that time. I have contacted the insurance company because they require a pre-authorization and detailed report from the doctor before they will approve the unscheduled eye exam. They must also pre-approve the new glasses which will, hopefully, permit her to see clearly again, as well as whatever else may be necessary to counter the vision-related side effects.

The end result of today's experience—yes, all in one day—was that she did not get a treatment and the entire program is set back at least a week. We will know better what to expect after we hear from the oncologist's office tomorrow.

Thanks to everyone for keeping us in their thoughts and prayers. We know they help.

Earle & Judy

No tidbit of good news is too minute to report. We were taking comfort from whatever source it came to us. This was one of those times.

Sunday, August 31, 2008

There is no big update to report, but there has been a development that I feel is important enough to share.

As you know from previous updates, one of the occurrences causing considerable concern has been the blurring of Judy's vision. There have been certain ways that we have been checking this on our own. One of the devices we have been using to monitor Judy's ability to see has been the time readout on the cable box. For the past week, Judy has not been able to discern the time display. Tonight, she announced that she was able to read the time. This is by no means an official determination, but it seems to be a step in the right direction. Until we see the doctor for the scheduled appointment on Tuesday, we are taking this to be a positive sign and considering it to be good news.

As I just said, Judy has a treatment planned for Tuesday. I'll be sending an update following that.

As always, our thanks to everyone for their continued thoughts and prayers, we feel they help.

Earle & Judy

Judy's Journey

It's amazing how much disruption to their lives humans can tolerate and still consider the situation normal. Here, the reference is made to the "normal degree of tiredness" and the now-accepted impairment to the sense of taste. How can this, even remotely, be thought of as "normal"? Regardless, here is that very observation.

Wednesday, September 3, 2008

This week's routine Monday treatment was disrupted by the Labor Day Holiday. I take full responsibility for the delay of an additional day in getting this update out. Sorry.

This treatment was the second of the double-dose chemotherapies. When we arrived for the appointment, Judy passed the initial exam. The white count was good and they were encouraged that her vision was showing signs of recovery. Her vision has continued to improve and we hope to close that door on Friday when she sees her ophthalmologist again.

The treatment went smoothly. Judy held up like the trooper that she is. The side effects seem to be pretty much limited to what has come to be thought of as the "normal degree of tiredness." The lack of taste continues to be an annoying side effect and makes for some disappointing meals. Her spirits remain high and we are both encouraged by the progress to date.

Thanks to everyone for your continued thoughts and prayers. We are certain that they help.

Earle & Judy

Although short, this personal message from Judy to her close friends is an indication of how arduous this fight actually is. She is so exhausted that she is warning her friends it will be some time before she is up to sending out any additional messages.

The content was so typical of Judy. No matter how badly she felt, she was still concerned about others.

Saturday, September 6, 2008

I wanted to let you know this has really knocked me on my butt this week. I am sick. If you don't hear from me, don't worry. I've been sleeping as much as I can lately. My body really hurts. I will drop you a line when I have the energy.

Judy

Humor played an enormous part in our being able to deal with the situation and a little of that shows up here. There are other admissions here that are disturbing though. They seem to have been a long time in coming.

Judy's acknowledgement that she was experiencing a significant level of pain and is asking for help for the first time is just a tiny indication of how overwhelmed she felt. Here, she also mentions a major problem that plagued her throughout the entire time she battled this disease as she struggled with an unrelenting pain in her hands and feet called neuropathy. (How all these medical terms found their way into our everyday conversations is, in itself, nothing short of amazing.)

The long-resisted admission related to her inability to continue working much longer is reluctantly mentioned here as well. Judy often commented that she had what she considered a dream job. She loved both the job and her fellow employees. She had a strong working relationship with her supervisors as well. The simple truth is that she considered those with whom she worked her second family. It was a feeling that was fully reciprocated.

Tuesday, September 9, 2008

Yesterday, Judy had her single dose treatment of Herceptin. It was noted that her white count was down so she was given a booster to bring it up. That's the shot which usually catches up with her by Wednesday and results in exhaustion for a few days thereafter.

She has finally admitted that she could use some help with pain management and accepted a prescription that will, hopefully, provide some relief. It has also been noted that since the start of treatment she has lost five pounds. This, in itself, does not raise any red flags, but bears watching. FYI—we would NOT recommend this as a weight loss program to anyone wanting to lose a few pounds!

Judy seemed to get a good night's rest last night and has been sleeping better the last few days. It has become apparent to her that she will be unable to continue working much longer. She has started the paperwork required to take the available medical leave. More on this as the process unfolds.

All is as well as can be reasonably expected. Judy's spirits are high and she still has a positive attitude. The medical folks remain encouraged by her progress. We are certain that all your thoughts and prayers are a big help.

Thank you one and all.

Earle & Judy

Monday, September 15, 2008

Today was Judy's day for the double treatment. In addition, both of her blood counts were low. She got an injection for the red count today and will get the one for the white count tomorrow. That's the shot that knocks her off her feet for much of the rest of the week. I expect that she will be keeping a low profile this week.

Perhaps it is a good thing that she is no longer working. She can now get all the rest that her body so desperately needs.

We are closing in on the final weeks of this round of chemo. We aren't 100% sure how things will go from here, but anticipate sitting down with the surgeon soon. Judy is still able to maintain a positive attitude and we are confident that one day we will be able to put this all behind us.

Again, thank you for all your prayers and thoughts. There is no doubt that they are a source of inner strength and we are sure they help.

Earle & Judy

Tuesday, September 23, 2008

Judy had her next to last chemotherapy treatment today. This was the single dose round. As anticipated, it went well. Both blood counts were good and, thankfully, no additional weight loss has been noted at this time. The P.A. handled the pretreatment exam. All went well.

The P.A. informed Judy that it would take four to six weeks after completion of the last treatment for the onset of any return of her sense of taste and for the tingling in the fingers and feet to begin to fade. She is definitely looking forward to that.

Judy is adjusting to not working. She is getting some much needed rest now. She is able to take a nap during the day whenever she needs to. The additional rest has made a big difference this week. She is more alert when she is awake. She seems to be stronger and functioning better too.

There is nothing unusual to report, but we are continually encouraged by the progress she is making. Next week, the big treatment is scheduled for Tuesday. The final consultation with the doctor will be on

Monday. We are hoping to have more details following that doctor's appointment.

Thanks to all for your continued thoughts and prayers. They have been the source of much comfort through these last few weeks.

Earle & Judy

The primary element of the treatment protocol has been completed. The critical chemotherapy requirements have been met and all that remains in that respect is the continued administration of the maintenance medication—Herceptin. This has been a huge hurdle to surmount. We were both encouraged by her having attained this milestone.

We were ready and anxious to get on with the next phase—the surgical treatment. Although this step is a key stumbling block for many in this situation, Judy and I had discussed this anticipated segment of the treatment plan extensively. Thankfully, we were now capable of putting all of the pieces into perspective. Through our exhaustive talks, we had finally reached a level of acceptance which aided us in acknowledging the necessity of the procedure. We could now accept its inevitability without the morbid fear that many people experience when confronted with the prospect of a mastectomy.

This too, we faced together—as a couple who remained committed to one another, in good times and bad.

Judy's Journey

Tuesday, September 30, 2008

We have reached a major milestone in this repetitive pattern of "something new every time we turn around." Judy has had her final chemotherapy treatment. ***YEAH TEAM!!!!***

She still has to have a year of Herceptin, but that is the milder drug that is not considered chemo. It is a lot less toxic and much more tolerable.

The oncologist's visit yesterday was encouraging. The doctor listed a number of possible side effects that Judy avoided by adhering to the prescribed measures established "to minimize the patient's level of discomfort." He said that she had "tolerated" the treatments well, observing that she had only lost five pounds through the entire process. He further indicated that the only residual side effect remaining—the tingling in the hands and feet—would likely go away in time. The loss of taste is expected to return as the Taxol wears off—probably in 4-6 weeks. He informed her that she can now anticipate new hair growth and expect the low energy levels to begin to fade. In other words, physically, she can expect to return to normal.

The next step will be to sit down with Dr. P., the surgeon, and find out what she proposes. That appointment is scheduled for this Thursday. It appears obvious that they don't want to waste any time in proceeding to the next level of treatment. We aren't sure if there is a medical reason for the urgent advancement, but we appreciate it. Once we are in the "groove," we would like to continue the progress rather than be forced to endure a holding pattern of wait - wait - wait.

All is as well as can be expected. Spirits are still high and we are both certain that all your thoughts and prayers have helped to get us to this point.

Thanks to all.

Earle & Judy

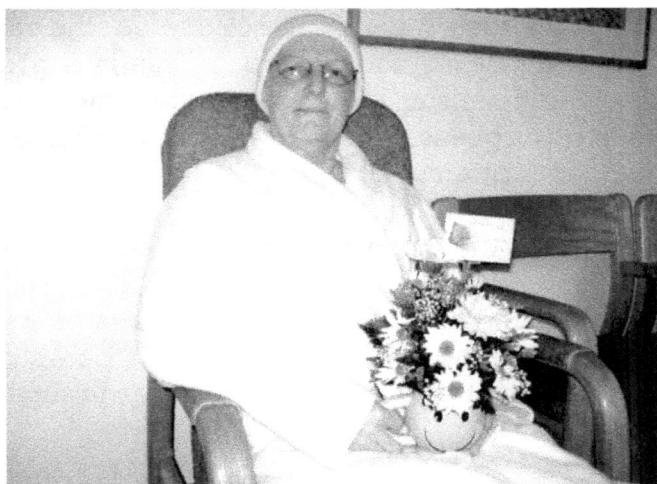

Judy reached her first major milestone — the completion of the critical pre-surgical chemotherapy.

Judy's Journey

Thursday, October 2, 2008

We have just returned from the initial consultation with the surgeon. The meeting went well and was quite informative.

We—all three of us—have agreed on the next step to take. First, the surgeon will contact the oncologist to discuss the results of the chemotherapy. She will then schedule a PET scan to assess the "whole body" condition. Following that, she plans to order an MRI to get a better picture of how the chemo has affected the original tumor in the breast.

When all of the tests have been conducted, the surgeon will meet with the "Tumor Board." This is a group of physician specialists who convene monthly for consultative purposes. They brainstorm specific cases and treatment options.

Following that consultation, we will meet again to review and discuss all of the treatment recommendations and decide which course of action to take. In all likelihood, the choices will be—surgery, radiation, or "wait and see"—or some combination of these.

We got the impression that the surgeon was more than "just pleased" with the results of the chemo. She actually seemed to be a little surprised that the tumors had responded to the chemo as well as they did. She indicated that she believed that our early action and the immediate medical intervention, when the condition was first detected, were pivotal factors in producing the excellent results we are seeing now from the chemo. We take this to be encouraging.

We still wholeheartedly believe that the ongoing thoughts and prayers from all of you have been a contributing factor as well. Our heartfelt thanks to each and every one of you once again.

Earle & Judy

> This personal message is from Judy to Lynda, her closest friend from school. In fact, Lynda was her Matron of Honor when we were married. This note details why Judy wasn't able to invite her to stop by for a visit. For Judy to have declined this opportunity to socialize with her best friend, she had to be seriously affected by the side effects of the treatments. Though significantly challenged, her positive attitude shines through true to form.

Saturday, October 4, 2008

Sorry I wasn't up for company today. This has not been a good week for me, but at least I know from here on it will get better. I really have problems with my feet and hands; so bad that I do not sleep well. When I am feeling better, we will get together on one of your days off.

I hope all is well with you. I do miss you.

Judy

Judy's Journey

This may well be the lengthiest personal message Judy sent out to her friends. It was penned on Sunday, Columbus Day, following the accident which she so eloquently describes—at my expense. Clearly, she was anxious to tell her friends of my incredible clumsiness. A touch of humor comes through as well.

What neither of us knew at the time was that this incident would turn out to be a true blessing in disguise. This will become readily apparent in future updates.

Sunday, October 12, 2008

You know the saying, "When it rains, it pours." Well, I think Earle and I have a hurricane over our heads this year.

Earle and his brother were taking down a pool deck today for our friend. Earle took a bad fall and I ended up driving him to the emergency room. You know [me] the one with the numb feet [and] hands and fuzzy eyesight!!

We spent about three hours in the emergency room. It appears he may have a fractured wrist. He has to set up an appointment tomorrow with the orthopedic doctor. He will [then] make the determination as to how badly it is injured. Earle also hurt his back when he landed.

He is out of work until the doctor says he can [go] back. I have him sitting in his new chair; a birthday present which was delivered yesterday. The chair has a vibrator and heat in it so he is comfortable at the moment. The arm is in a splint and he has to keep ice on it. You know he is in good hands with me taking care of him. What a pair we make! I wanted to let you know how our day was; I sure hope your day was a lot better.

Judy

Time continues to pass and we are still running tests. Based on the initial urgency stressed during the surgical consult, we thought the process would have moved ahead much more quickly than this. However, we accept the fact that everything which is being done is to insure Judy's safety and well-being during the treatment.

This update went out shortly after the Columbus Day weekend during which I experienced the little misadventure Judy alluded to in the preceding message. As improbable as it sounds, I fell—while standing flat on the ground—and broke my wrist. This has furnished some "friends" with an inexhaustible source of chiding at my expense.

It certainly complicated our schedule. In the larger sense, however, as I mentioned earlier, it was a true blessing in disguise. As a result of my clumsiness, I was on disability for the next three months. This made it possible for me to be on hand to provide all the necessary transportation and to be available to be by Judy's side during the next big phase of her treatment plan: the surgery.

Perhaps it is true; all things do happen for a reason—
we just aren't always privy to the plan. I am reminded
of a spiritual reference that teaches us that "all things
work together for good to them that love the Lord, to
them, who are the called according to His purpose."
(Romans 8:28, KJV). Friends later shared that this
scripture had certainly crossed their minds at the time
as well.

Tuesday, October 14, 2008

It's been two weeks since Judy's last chemo session.
She is still receiving the Herceptin. Though not actually
considered chemotherapy, it is a maintenance
medication intended to suppress tumor generation.
The Herceptin administration is to continue for a year.
The other side effects are slowly wearing off. Some
taste is returning, but the "biggie," the numbness and
tingling in the hands and feet, remains quite prevalent
and troublesome. Judy still doesn't have to shave either
(but I'm not sure if she considers that as a side effect or
a benefit). She remains quite tired, but has been able to
manage her schedule so that she can keep up with the
Red Sox.

She is scheduled for a PET scan tomorrow. We expect
she will go for an MRI after that. Once those tests have
been completed, we should receive some more
definitive information as to what course of action we will
be pursuing. In the interim, she is avoiding exposure to
any possible infection and getting plenty of much-
needed rest.

As an aside; I got the word from the orthopedic surgeon today that my misadventure on Sunday did, in fact, result in a broken wrist. I have been "casted" (no, not in a play) and will be laid up for an undetermined amount of time. I will get a progress report on November 5th, but won't know anything conclusive until then. It appears that I am destined to send out double updates from now on.

We are having some fun now.

Earle & Judy

> This next update describes one of the emotional high points which had been glaringly absent for some time during our strange medical odyssey. At last, some positive news. In addition to the good news, we now have a clearer picture of the next phase of Judy's treatment.

> Finally, we are moving forward. Advancement is an element that has been frustratingly absent recently—at least from our perspectives—as we observe and actually "live" the process. It feels like we've been "running in place" for a long time.

> My condition is unchanged—my arm is still in a cast—but I am hopefully providing enough help to offset the extra work my disability creates. We are dealing with the situation as best we can and enjoying each other's company throughout the day. We joke that this is our dress rehearsal for when I retire. Although we make light of this, it is, in fact, an excellent window into what to expect in the foreseeable future.

Judy's Journey

Friday, October 17, 2008

We received some news today from the Oncology Center and the surgeon at the Women's Health Center. When Judy's doctor called to speak with Judy, I took the call since Judy was having a treatment at the time. From her tone, I could tell that she was very positive. She was quite obviously eager to speak to Judy—so much so, that she gave me her personal cell number and instructions to "have Judy call just as soon as she came home."

When Judy returned the call, we learned that the results of the PET scan were in. They came back better than anyone ever dared to hope. They revealed that all affected areas are clear and clean! There were no active cancer cells in evidence!! This is unequivocally the best possible news we could have received. We are elated to hear this.

Now we are able to move on to the next step. We now, in fact, know what the next step is. Surgery is scheduled for November 6th. The surgery will include a mastectomy and the removal of some of the lymph nodes from beneath the left arm. After the surgery has been completed and the surgical site healed, there will be a round of radiation. We have been told that any reconstructive surgery will take place about a year after the original operation, as adequate time for healing must be allowed before attempting that procedure.

We are thrilled with the outcome of the chemo. Though more than a little apprehensive, we are looking forward to taking the next step in this journey, so we can speak of it in the past tense.

Of minor note, I am in a cast for a fractured left wrist as noted in earlier updates. We make quite a pair. After doing the math, we figure that between the two of us we add up to about two-thirds of a person. We are making the best of it and facing the challenge of scheduling our lives around doctor visits.

As always, we thank you all for your most generous thoughts and prayers. We are certain that they have helped get us to where we are at now.

Thanks to all.

Earle & Judy

Finally, we are making encouraging progress. The plan is coming together and we feel like we are moving forward. Specific dates have been set for the pre-op procedures, as well as the date for the surgery.

We no longer have to endure uncertainties and anticipation—we have a target to focus on.

At this time, I am still on the "Disabled List." I sincerely hope that I am not weighing Judy down with extra work because of it.

Mention is made of our new chairs. Judy had decided that she wanted to replace our old couch with two recliners, so we each picked out the chair of our dreams and had them delivered. In retrospect, this turned out to be an extraordinarily, well-timed decision; soon, Judy's chair would become her 24-hour haven.

I don't know if she anticipated this occurrence or if it just worked out that way, but the addition of the new chairs was timely indeed—for both of us.

Wednesday, October 22, 2008

Progress is being made in Judy's treatment. We now have firm dates for the pre-op consultation and the actual surgery.

On November 6th, we will be meeting with Dr. P., the surgeon, for the "pep talk" and pre-op procedures, EKG, etc. The surgery has been booked for November 13th which coincides with the six-week anniversary of Judy's last chemo treatment.

The surgery is scheduled to be a single mastectomy of the left breast and removal of some of the lymph nodes from her left arm. We asked about the advisability of including the right side as well. *(This is now being done more commonly as a preventive measure, particularly when there is increased breast cancer risk in a patient.)* The oncology specialist has advised us that it is best to take care of what we know must be dealt with now. Additional delays would likely result because further tests would be required to justify the removal of the other side. We agree to the wisdom of taking this one step at a time.

The rationale, that is the pressing for immediacy, is that this type of cancer is so aggressive. We need to get this step behind us and then remain vigilant in monitoring any possible relapse. Barring anything unforeseen, Judy is expected to be hospitalized for only one night. We are pleased the stay will be short. We had anticipated that the hospital recovery time would be longer.

As the days go by, Judy is showing continued improvements and recovery from the side effects of the last chemo. Her hands and feet still ache, but are getting better. She continues to experience a decreased energy level, but is keeping as active as she is able. Her new chair is getting a workout.

I'm still unsure if my being home is helpful or not. I'd like to think it is, but being one-handed—while my broken wrist is in a cast and healing—limits my ability to contribute to the daily tasks. I do what I can though. We now share everything—yes, even those afternoon naps. My new chair is working out well also.

Our heartfelt thanks go out to everyone for keeping us in their thoughts and prayers. We are certain they help.

We send our best to each and every one of you.

Earle & Judy

As we see here, Judy continues to keep her friends up-to-date on my patient status. She even went so far as to send pictures of me in my injured state. All kidding aside, I really didn't mind, especially since it gave her a new topic of discussion and something to take her mind off of her own trials.

Wednesday, November 5, 2008

Earle went to the doctor's today to have his wrist checked. It seems to be healing. He has a new cast and has to return on November 26th to have it checked again. He is experimenting with colors. The first cast was blue, the second red.

He is still unable to return to work.

Judy

Thursday, November 6, 2008

This has been a busy time leading up to the scheduled surgery next week. Judy had the Herceptin treatment last Friday—Halloween. Those treatments will be continuing for the next year. As mentioned previously, these are a maintenance type of treatment. While it is administered like the chemo, it is not considered a chemo treatment. Thankfully, it is a quick procedure and is free of side effects.

Wednesday, I had my appointment to assess the healing progress of my wrist fracture. It went well, the x-ray showed signs of healing. At this time, it would seem that no surgery will be needed. The wrist was casted again. I will go back in three weeks for another check. I am now sporting a bright red cast.

Today, Judy and I had an educational appointment in preparation for the upcoming pre-op and post-op procedures. We had a thorough initiation as to what to expect leading up to the surgery and what the primary concerns after the operation will be. The meeting was informative and answered a lot of our questions.
Following that interview, Judy completed her pre-op tests and paperwork. We are as ready as we can be for the next step in the extensive process focused on beating this insidious disease.

Her surgery is scheduled for 10:00 a.m., on Thursday the 13th. A two-hour procedure is anticipated. She is expected to remain in the hospital overnight. Judy's mindset is positive and her attitude is that of someone ready to move on. We are prepared, ready, and confident that we are on track to achieve a successful outcome.

We have to thank each and every one of you for your ongoing support and prayers. We are certain that you have all contributed to Judy's progress to date and we appreciate the continued good thoughts.

The next update will be after the surgery.

Thanks again to all.

Earle & Judy

Judy's Journey

The long anticipated day of surgery has finally arrived—surprisingly, without the now-anticipated delays or change of plans. We are intent to put this step behind us. As much as we have talked about it and have absolutely no doubt as to the necessity of this surgical procedure, being on the threshold of the operation has brought some pangs of apprehension and anxiety to both of us. Once again, Judy's positive and pragmatic attitude was revealed as she bid me farewell with a smile. I assured her that I would be waiting for her when she came out.

A passing reference is made here to my limited computer skills. It should be noted that Judy was my instructor in all things computer-related. With her temporary incapacitation, I now had to fly solo for the first time. Now, in addition to the operation, I could focus on being nervous about something else—but maybe that was a bit of a blessing in disguise as well.

Thursday, November 13, 2008

I'm in charge of running both computers tonight, so if things look a little different that's the reason. The fact that I had to start this in "Word" and then transfer it to the body of the e-mail message put my computer skills to their maximum test.

Earle

I am starting this while in the waiting room at the hospital. We came in about 8:00 this morning and went through all the pre-op procedures.

There is a lot of checking and double-checking. I can't understand how those botched surgeries that you hear about on the news can possibly happen.

Everything went fine. They used Judy's port for the IV, which worked out well. All of the involved players stopped by for their final check-in: the OR nurse, the anesthesiologist, and the surgeon. They wheeled her into the OR right on time. Then, still on schedule, about noon, Dr. P., the surgeon, came into the waiting room and told us—our daughter was with me—that the operation had gone well. Everything that could be determined visually was positive. We will be advised of the test results at the next appointment. We are scheduled to see Dr. P. on Tuesday, the 18th. We will find out any additional information then. The drains will be removed at that time as well.

It's getting close to the time we were told she would be transferred to the room, so I'll finish this at home tonight.

(Later)
OK, it's almost 6:00 p.m. and I am now home. Everything went without a hitch. Judy regained consciousness earlier than expected and we were settled in her room by 1:30 p.m. She was awake, alert, and aware of her surroundings. I stayed with her until about 4:30 this afternoon; long enough to see that she was settled. She actually threw me out so she could take a nap before the Patriots game tonight—GO PATS!

Judy was able to get out of bed and travel to the "powder room" under her own steam. That, in itself, has to be a good thing. When I left, she still had an IV. It did not contain any meds, but was a precautionary measure to be sure she didn't get dehydrated after the operation. She still had the leg wraps on as well. *(These are intended to keep blood from pooling in the legs—and prevent blood clots from forming—following surgery.)* I expect they will come off sometime tonight.

While I was there, they brought her a diet tray of clear liquids. In case you don't know, that consists of some real tasty stuff. The main course was chicken broth, yum! There was Jell-O, two kinds of juice, and sorbet. Nothing to write home about, but I assure you the tray went back empty! The doctor's order was that she could advance to a full liquid diet and then to regular food as she was able to tolerate the changes.

While I was there, I got a real-life lesson in what is needed to clear the drains. There are two and I am confident that I will be able to handle the task. Since I am still home (recuperating from that fall I took in October) there will be no need for a Visiting Nurse.

If all goes as planned—and at this point, I see no reason why it won't—she should be home and settled in her La-Z-Boy sometime tomorrow.

We have an appointment for next Tuesday afternoon to see the surgeon in her office and have the drains removed. Everything seems to be going according to plan at this time.

I can't emphasize how much all of your thoughts and prayers have helped us get to this stage. Thank you one and all for everything.

Earle & Judy

This was the personal message Judy sent out to her friends on the day that she came home following the surgery. It is interesting to compare the different points of view as each of us reported about the events of the same day.

Friday, November 14, 2008

I wanted to let you know I'm home. I'm doing just fine, a little sore but not bad. I have only taken one pain pill and that was last night when my Patriots were struggling!!

I will not be moving out of my chair for a few days. I am not supposed to lift anything or use my left arm much.

Earle did a great job draining my tubes. The nurse was very proud of him, as was I. He will have his hands (hand?) full with me this weekend. He has to help me get dressed and make sure I am eating and drinking like I am supposed to. I am so lucky to have him home with me. The broken wrist has worked out in our favor.

When I left the hospital, I was dressed all in pink. I made the nurses smile because I was so color coordinated. They said I was a great patient and they wish they had more patients like me: never a complaint and I only rang the buzzer when I needed help to the restroom. If they only knew! I'm not always good—just when I'm out in public.

Thanks for all your support, we read all your comments that you write. You are such great support to us. I still have a long way to go, but at least we have moved up one more step in the process.

Judy

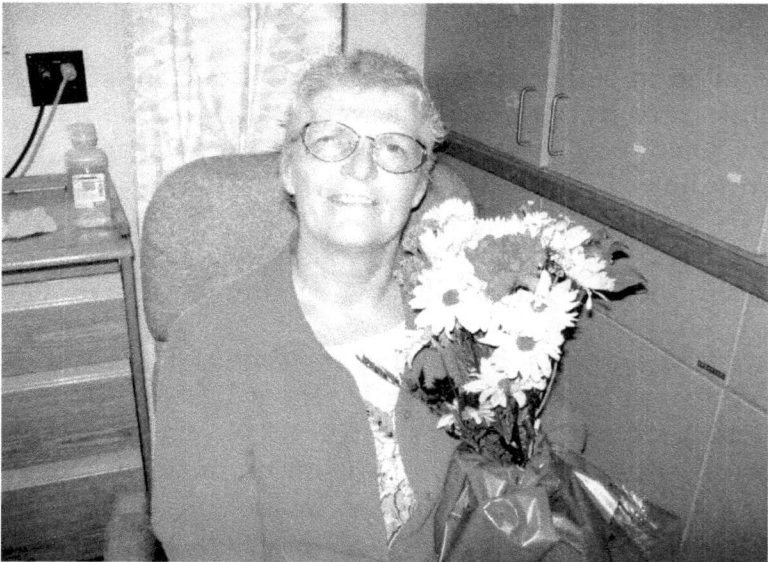

Judy, dressed in pink and ready for discharge following her surgery.

What follows is the update which I sent out on the same subject.

Friday, November 14, 2008

The situation changed rapidly from last night to today. Last night for supper, Judy had the "beloved broth and Jell-O" special.

This morning, it was pancakes and the fixings. She called me at 8:00 a.m. to chat, and again at 8:30 or so, to say "Come get me!" The doctor was in during breakfast. He looked her over and pronounced her fit to go home.

I, of course, dashed in and in a mere 2 1/2 hours we were out of there. We got out just before the official "check out time." (To which nobody pays a bit of attention!)

Things worked out well, though. I was there when the nurse came in for the final review and checks. I actually "gloved up" and did the drain maintenance with the nurse's supervision. This is the task which I have to perform for the next few days until we go to the post-operative appointment on Tuesday. I was confident before, but now I am certain I can do the procedure. The nurse was kind enough to supply me with a box of gloves—more than enough to get us to Tuesday.

Judy is doing fine. She is almost pain-free. I expect that once she gets settled in her chair and doesn't have to move around so much, she should be OK.

Judy's Journey

The timing has worked out well, I'm still "adapting" to life with a cast and I am now able to do a little more. I can provide more help to Judy than what I was able to accomplish during those first few days. Once we get settled into a schedule, we'll be fine. We're both glad to be making progress and look forward to seeing this through to its completion.

Once again, our deepest thanks to everyone for your continued thoughts and prayers. Knowing that your support has been there for us, has been a great feeling. Thank you, thank you, and thank you.

Earle & Judy

Once again in a personal message, we get some insight into Judy's state of mind and her condition. Here, she relates her homecoming to her supervisor at work.

At this time, both of our mindsets are that when the treatments are concluded and after an appropriate period of recuperation, she will be returning to work. This objective is one of the targets which motivated Judy to maintain that progressive momentum.

Saturday, November 15, 2008

I wanted to let you know I'm home. A little sore but not bad; the hospital staff told me I was a very good patient and they wish they had more like me. If only they really knew, huh!!!! Earle drained my tubes and did a good job even though he only has the one hand. They were proud of him, as was I.

I won't be moving out of my chair for a few days. [I have] strict orders not to lift anything and not to use my left arm much.

Please say HELLO to everyone and let them know I miss them, especially all MY MEN!!!! I miss everyone so much!!!

Judy

Tuesday, November 18, 2008

We have good news! One more step is now behind us.

We saw the surgeon today. She examined the site, as well as my meticulous chart of the drainage records, and determined that the drains were ready to be removed. They are, in fact, gone now. Judy has an arm exercise to do in order to prevent the muscles on her left side from getting tight or atrophying.

Then, the doctor gave us the best news we've had in a week: as of tomorrow, Judy has the official OK to take an actual shower. This is a major step forward at this point.

We go back next week for another follow-up. I'm not sure how long this will be necessary or how many follow-ups will be required, but for now, it's enough to know that we are moving forward. **Oh Boy!!**

Judy's Journey

Thanks to everyone for your continued support, good thoughts, and prayers.

Earle & Judy

> At this juncture, the news which follows was the single biggest announcement we had made to this point. We were, in fact, at the pinnacle of that virtual roller coaster. There was giddiness all around. We were not certain how—if at all—this would affect the prescribed program we were following, but at the time, we were overjoyed at the good news.
>
> We made sure that we thanked our supporters for their contribution. Regardless of what anyone else may have thought, we were convinced that they were as much a part of this celebration as we were and they all deserved some credit too.

Wednesday, November 19, 2008

I realize this is a bit "on the heels" of yesterday's update, but this is so good that we just have to share the news. The surgeon called today with the results from the pathologist. Apparently the two rounds of chemo were so effective that there were _**no signs of any remaining cancer.**_ In fact, the surgeon related to us that the pathologist inquired first, if this was truly a cancer patient. When she assured him that it was, he asked if the tissue specimen that she had sent him, was actually from the affected breast. The surgeon was so excited with the results, she was nearly giddy. She said the pathologist told her that he had good news for her—unless she made a mistake—and asked her to sit down before he shared the results. The surgeon was so eager to share the news with Judy and me that she called us just as soon as she had hung up from getting the pathology report.

We aren't certain yet how this translates in the full scope of the treatment plan. We don't know if this means that radiation won't be needed or if anything else that has been planned will change. At this point, we are simply thrilled to be so blessed to have reached this stage in the process and to have received such a positive report.

We send heartfelt thanks to each and every one of you for your continued support, your good thoughts, and prayers. We are sure this confirms what we have said since the start—they have all helped.

Earle & Judy

> This is a routine, straightforward update. It recounts the progress Judy is making in her recovery, but also highlights the rapidity with which the process continues to move forward. Before we are completely finished with the surgery stage, we were already having consultations concerning the next stage: radiation.
>
> All of this is happening while I am still on the "disabled list" with the broken wrist. Being home during these two phases of the treatment was the "blessing in disguise" which I mentioned earlier. The upcoming radiation treatments are going to be intense and could

have presented a true logistical nightmare, but my unexpected availability averted any potential problems in this area. How many times have we heard that "God moves in mysterious ways"? We consider this development proof of that observation.

There is also mention of some e-mail delivery glitches in this update. These plagued our news delivery system, off and on, throughout the entire time. We never discovered the source of some of the problems. Undoubtedly, my limited computer abilities probably played a part in the ongoing difficulties.

Wednesday, November 26, 2008

This has been a busy week in our house. Monday, Judy had her tri-weekly appointment for the Herceptin treatment. These will continue for a year from when they started. She should finish sometime next July.

Tuesday, we had the second follow-up with the surgeon, Dr. P. She checked the incision area and removed the surgical tape that was still in place. The site is healing well. There is no sign of infection or of any accumulation of fluids.

The surgeon told us that she had used a new harmonic scalpel in the operation and she was pleased with the outcome. (*Harmonic scalpels are surgical instruments which use ultrasonic energy to decrease blood loss by permitting an incision to be made while simultaneously cauterizing the tissue edges with a single multi-function device. This reduces the time required for a surgical procedure to be completed. It also diminishes the risk of heat-related tissue damage. Traditional cautery is more time-consuming and increases the risk of heat injury and burns to adjacent tissue because it uses thermal energy, in the form of heat, to seal leaking blood vessels.)*

We have an appointment with the radiologist for the introduction and instructions for the next step which will be the radiation phase. We expect that to be a daily treatment for five weeks concluding by the end of January. It would seem that we are, indeed, seeing that proverbial "light at the end of the tunnel."

I had my second follow-up for my wrist and I am now sporting my third cast. This one is a bright green to keep in the spirit of the season. My doctor found something suspicious in the X-ray and has scheduled a CT scan to get a better picture of what is going on. I won't have a definitive answer on the status of my healing until after the scan comes back and he can read it. We should know more in about a week or so.

As always, we thank you all for the continued thoughts and prayers. We are now more certain than ever that they all help.

Earle & Judy

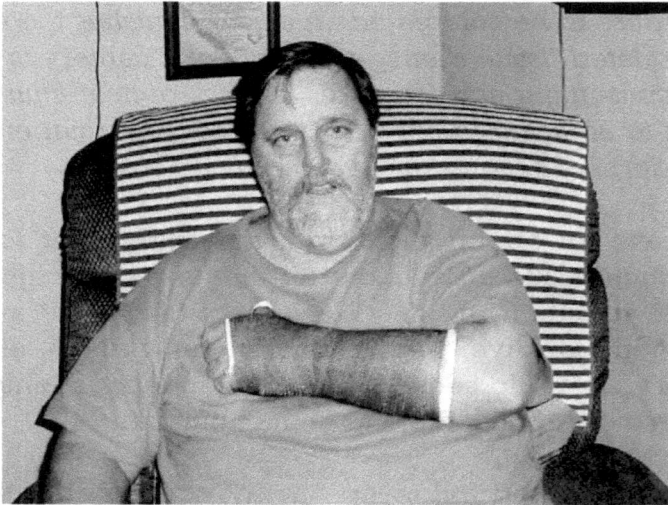

Earle, now sporting his third cast—Christmas Green!

Saturday, December 6, 2008

Sorry this is a little late. I should have sent it out yesterday. Judy's condition continues to improve. Her stamina is increasing and her hair growth is returning. We see the radiologist on Monday to find out what the schedule will be for the radiation treatments. That will be the last part of the treatment protocol. After that, if all goes well, there will just be the Herceptin every three weeks.

My situation continues to improve as well. Last Thursday, the doctor read the CT scan and determined that the original bone fracture was healed. The one that he was concerned about was, in fact, not damaged. Consequently, I am no longer in a cast and I will be doing "home therapy" for the next two weeks. On the 17th, I will go back to see how far I have progressed and whether or not I will need further therapy.

Once again, thanks to all for keeping us in your thoughts and prayers. We are sure that they have helped get us to this point.

Earle & Judy

This is perhaps the lengthiest update in the entire collection. In it, several subjects are covered, including a four-day power outage that challenged our abilities to cope under stressful circumstances. We passed the test. This rite of passage bolstered our confidence and gave us the assurance that we would be able to handle any situation which confronted us in the future.

The remainder of the message chronicles our progress toward the next step in the treatment protocol: radiation. It also recounts Judy's first experience with the art of tattooing, an encounter she would not soon forget.

Monday, December 15, 2008

First, let me assure everyone that you have not been forgotten. In case you had not heard, we have just emerged from a mini Ice Age. Last Thursday, it rained all day and night. When the temperature dropped below freezing, everything above the ground became completely coated in ice. The tree population took a huge hit. The power lines took it even harder. We lost power at 11:05 p.m. Thursday. Judy was scheduled for her first radiation therapy session on Friday morning, but when it became clear that leaving the yard was not an option, we settled in to address the priorities at home.

For us, the first thing to check after a heavy rain is the sump hole in the cellar. It turned out that the water in the hole was at the top and ready to overflow at any minute. This called for the emergency power supply. We broke out the generator that we had purchased ten years prior, following the big ice storm in '98. Since it was last pressed into service two years earlier, it has been collecting dust in the garage. I expected a bit of trouble getting it started. I quickly expended all of the energy I could muster with no result—remember, I was still challenged by the fact that my left arm had been immobilized in a cast until very recently. Our son, Chuck also tried to start it when he stopped by later. By the time Chuck left, it quickly became clear that professional help was going to be needed.

In the meantime, we turned to our small camp generator. It's a low wattage unit that would run the pump, but not much more. It started hard—but it did start—and handled the water in the sump just fine.

You should have seen Judy and me trying to load the "new" primary generator into the truck, given our combined limitations. But load it we did, and made it to the Honda shop in Manchester by about 3:00 p.m.—they close at 6:00.

The entire place was awash in generators. While he was cashing out another customer and before I had said a word, the service manager quickly identified my problem. To say that he had seen this problem before was an understatement. An hour later, following one carburetor clean-out, a lesson on how to properly shut down a generator, and $80, the unit was as good as new.

We returned home about 6:00 p.m. or so, connected the proper wires, fired up the unit on two pulls, threw the breakers on the Gen-Tran switch, and we had the necessities of life: heat, running water, hot water, as well as power to the freezer, refrigerator, and a few lights. The unit ran non-stop right up until Monday morning when the power was restored.

This storm has been an experience I would not want to repeat soon, but we made it through. We were also able to provide heat and shelter to my brother and his wife as well. I understand they are shopping for a generator as I compose this message.

Back to the original message, we have met with the doctor who will be Judy's radiologist, Dr. K. He seems very nice and extremely thorough. He already knew the particulars of Judy's case and, in fact, told us things we had forgotten. He had actually sat on the "Tumor Board" (which had originally determined the best course of treatment in Judy's case). He had also already been in contact with all of her other doctors.

He has ordered a course of physical therapy to strengthen the muscles in her arm. The PT and endurance training will promote her ability to regain sufficient range of motion to enable her to maintain the position necessary for the next course of treatment.

He also ordered some additional tests before starting the radiation treatment. The tests are needed to ensure that there has been no undetected spread of the cancer before initiating the radiation process. The treatment program itself will last for six weeks and will be administered five days a week if everything remains on schedule.

Judy's first physical therapy appointment is tomorrow. Later this week, she will return to the radiology department for a "positioning" session. It is our understanding that this consists of making some markings to insure precise, identical positioning of the radiation device to accurately deliver the radiation beam. They will also make something called a mask to help in the positioning as well.

Judy continues to show consistent progress in all other areas of treatment. We remain highly hopeful for a successful outcome at the end of the prescribed protocol.

We also value the continued thoughts and prayers from all of you. We feel they have helped get us to this point and look forward to more good reports in the future. Thank you one and all.

Earle & Judy

With the holidays approaching, we sent this note. It is not really an update, but something to let our growing support network know that we acknowledge and appreciate their dedication and well wishes.

The e-card was Judy's forte. She was an expert at finding and sending cards like this. Though she had been unable to manage this herself, there is no doubt that she was advising me as to how to accomplish the task of including it in the message. (The link that opens an e-Christmas card was included in the original message.)

Saturday, December 20, 2008

This is just a quick note to thank you all for keeping us in your hearts and prayers. We are certain that the support from all of you has helped get us to where we are today. We are truly grateful.

The link below should open up a Christmas card which we would like you to accept from us. (Link omitted.)

Thank you for being there for us.

Earle & Judy

As 2008 draws to a close, we have seen, done, and experienced a great deal in our attempts to keep this hideous monster called cancer at bay. We have seen what we can accomplish together as a team; we have done things which we would never have dreamed possible; and we have experienced the benefits of a medical community devoted to the treatment and care of patients such as Judy.

We have gained much from the fellowship of our many friends and family who have stood by us and supported us with heartfelt wishes and prayers. In addition to practical day-to-day logistical assistance, they have provided us with much spiritual support. We consider ourselves very blessed as 2008 comes to an end. We look forward to continuing the fight in the New Year and more importantly, to soundly defeating this foe.

Friday, December 26, 2008

As 2008 comes to a close, we hope you all had a Merry Christmas and are looking forward to a Happy New Year. We have some encouraging news to report.

Judy has had all the tests ordered by the radiologist. Everything came back normal. The scans included a new MRI of the head to confirm that no cancer had spread to the brain. This was a heightened concern because of the brain tumor she had dealt with almost six years ago. The test was a concern to us as well, but the films show no cancer in this area. This was welcome news indeed.

The worst thing that the assessments revealed was that Judy would need some physical therapy to regain the range of motion in her left arm. This is essential in order to be able to assume—and more importantly to maintain—the necessary position required during the radiation treatment.

Today was Judy's final therapy appointment. Now she just has to do some home exercises to ensure that she doesn't backslide by the time the treatment begins.

In addition, she had the "dry run" for the radiation. She has had the target dots tattooed on her to identify the specific treatment area. Though they are actual tattoos, they are just pinprick size dots. The experience has absolutely confirmed her previous opinion—she has NO desire to get any type of tattoo. In fact, she questions how anyone could actually want to go through the process. I explained that the majority of tattoos are the result of excessive partying and/or celebrating. They are usually applied at a time when there is a reduced awareness of pain. As she nodded thoughtfully, I could almost hear her thinking, "Another good reason to not drink."

As we progress in her treatment plan, it looks like she will be starting radiation shortly after the first of January. She is currently scheduled to complete the process sometime in the middle of February. At this point, we are looking forward to getting this step behind us and we are sure it will go well.

On another front, my recovery is progressing as well. I am one week into OT for my wrist; and PT for my back. The therapists are competent and I am comfortable dealing with them. I admit that I was somewhat dubious as to what they would be able to do, but after just one week I am now confident they have some good ideas about how to get me back to a level of function which will allow me to return to work. My appointments are scheduled through mid-January. I hope that will be sufficient as I am ready to return to a regular schedule.

As always, we want to thank everyone for your continued good thoughts and prayers. We are certain they have all helped to get us to this point.

Earle & Judy

2009

The New Year has started, but the same bumps in the road are trying to trip us up. This message is another indication of what we were coming to accept as the inevitable—the endless roller coaster ride that the treatment protocol would continue to take us on. Unfortunately, this was one of the many low points we were to endure.

If these disappointments affected Judy's positive—some might even say, enthusiastic—attitude, she never showed it. She always accepted the current situation with the outlook that "whatever was meant to be, would be." This view of the human condition served her well throughout her entire life. It was especially comforting at this time under these adverse conditions. I should also mention that to a great extent, Judy's characteristic strength and affirmative stance were an inspiration to me. They continually reinforced my own resolve to remain fully committed to her and to unconditionally support her decisions in the ongoing fight she was so valiantly waging. To be perfectly honest, her strength of character had been a source of steadfastness for me throughout our entire relationship.

Thursday, January 8, 2009

At this time, I should have been reporting to you that we have reached another milestone. Instead, I have to tell you that we have encountered another stumbling block.

Today was the day scheduled for Judy's first radiation treatment. It is a day we have been working toward for some time now. We arrived at the Radiology Center at the appointed time. When Judy went in for the procedure, they discovered an unusual rash that had mysteriously appeared the day before. It had now developed into a case of shingles. After a great deal of discussion and consultation with her bevy of doctors, it was decided to suspend the radiation and treat the shingles with Valtrex. Since they caught the malady at such an early stage, they are confident that they can successfully treat it. Unfortunately, this put everything else on hold. As it is now, she is scheduled to see the doctor on the 20th of January. It is hoped that the shingles will have subsided by then and that they will be able to proceed with the radiation.

This puts the six-week radiation timetable about a week and a half behind schedule. Understandably, we are disappointed, but we fully understand the importance of doing whatever it takes to ensure the best possible result from the radiation. Hopefully, we will have better news for you in the next update.

As always, thank you for keeping us in your thoughts and prayers. We do appreciate it.

Earle & Judy

Here, after nearly the entire month of January has passed, the update goes out that the radiation treatment schedule is now finally underway. The intensity of the treatments is starting to wear on Judy.

This message also reports the somewhat surprising news that I have finally returned to work. The rigors of returning to the ranks of the employed after a three-month hiatus, has motivated me to seriously look into my retirement options.

Friday, January 30, 2009

Sorry this has been so long in coming. A lot of little things have been happening and my time, suddenly, became no longer my own. That's a convoluted way of saying, "I've returned to work"—but we'll get to that later.

Judy's shingles have calmed down enough to start the radiation. She has almost two weeks of treatment sessions behind her and has about four weeks to go. The treatments are going well and creating only a minimum of side effects; predominately fatigue. She is still suffering from the lingering effects of the chemo in the form of numbness and pain in her feet. Her hands and fingers are improving, but her feet are still significantly impacted.

At some point in the last two weeks, the doctor also ordered a scan of the thyroid and "something" showed up. In order to determine the nature of this anomaly, Judy is scheduled to have a biopsy next week. The doctor doesn't seem overly concerned about this, but the biopsy will help resolve the nature of what the scan identified. If any action is required, it will take place after the radiation is completed.

The doctor told her that she could expect a sore throat soon because the radiation is being administered to a wider area than normal. This is required in order to insure the inclusion of all of the lymph nodes that were potentially affected. Unfortunately, this extended target area causes the esophagus to be irradiated and usually results in an extremely sore throat. To lighten the tone, we are now discussing what type of baby food she would like.

Judy continues to maintain a positive attitude, but the strain of the extended treatment is starting to wear on her. The ongoing bouts of fatigue have become quite bothersome as well, compelling us to curtail much in the way of activities beyond the necessary medical appointments. We apologize to anyone who has offered to visit. We have had no choice but to decline. When her energy level drops, it plummets so fast that sometimes even I am a little slow to pick up on it. Hopefully, things will improve after the radiation is completed.

From the other camp, my physical therapist and doctor both released me to return to work on the 19th of January. The company required me to see their doctor for a pre-return to work physical. I did that on Monday the 19th, and reported for work on Tuesday the 20th, after more than three months on the "Disabled List." I was lucky; the first day was a "1" on a scale of 1-10. It was the easiest possible day that it could have been.

When I returned home, however, I was so exhausted that I felt like I had been wrung out through a wringer. As soon as I was able to muster the energy, I accessed the pension website and checked my numbers to see how soon I could retire. I now have two light weeks behind me. My energy level is improving. I am confident that I will be able to return to my prior level of activity. The visit to the pension site was interesting enough that I have scheduled an appointment with the Pension Officer to get a firm handle on just what my options are. I think I'm going to be looking at two more years for the best deal, but I am going to find out.

As always, we want to thank everyone for their continued thoughts and prayers.

We are grateful for all the support. We are certain that you have all helped us get to where we are at.

Earle & Judy

> This next message is a short personal note from Judy to her immediate supervisors at work. At this point, we are all confident that she will soon be completing the course of treatment and be able to return to work.
>
> This goal has been a great motivator for Judy. It has inspired her to press on through the increasingly wearisome treatments.

Monday, February 9, 2009

I just got home from my radiation treatment and the doctor met with me today. My thyroid test came back cancer-free, I do have a problem with it [but we're] not sure what yet. They are going to keep an eye on it for the time being. The best news is; it is not cancerous, especially from the breast cancer.

My plan is to be back [to work] the first part of March. I don't finish treatment until around March 3rd. You know things change, but I plan on returning as soon as they sign the paper.

Earle will be sending out an update soon, but I wanted to let you know first what is happening.

Miss you all.

Judy

Next, the unpredictable nature of the disease and treatment process is confirmed again. An unexpected dilemma is indicated by an abnormal shortness of breath that hadn't been a problem in the past. This observation resulted in more impromptu tests and visits to the hospital, adding to the increasing strain of the continuing procedures. As indicated here, some of the continuing side effects are becoming increasingly bothersome and present a real concern.

A brief outline of my ongoing efforts at work is also mentioned here. My situation, however, is taking a backseat to the primary subject matter for which the updates were intended—to report on Judy's progress and condition as she traverses the unfamiliar waters of cancer treatment.

Monday, February 16, 2009

I realize it has been some time since the last update, but in truth: there was nothing to report. Everything was progressing as expected and all was going well. Today, that has changed a little.

Today was Judy's scheduled Herceptin treatment. Since today was also a holiday, I was available to take her to that session. In the pretreatment phase during the interview and exam by the P.A., the shortness of breath which Judy has been experiencing recently was discussed. The P.A. did some in-office tests including a brisk walk around the facility with an O^2 sensor on Judy's finger. All levels were normal and the blood work showed everything to be OK. The next step was to order some additional tests at the hospital. One of the tests, a CT scan, had to be done right away; another, the heart echocardiogram, is scheduled for Wednesday.

We expect that the test results will be forwarded to the radiologist. He will inform us of the outcome sometime this week. When we know more, we will pass it on.

Otherwise, things are going as well as can be expected. Judy is experiencing a great deal of fatigue due to the radiation. The pain in her feet (as a result of the chemotherapy) still bothers her. Though it is getting a little better, there is some concern due to its extended duration. We will continue to pursue answers from the doctors if it continues.

As an aside, I have been back to work for three weeks now. Work is slow, but this has provided me with a perfect opportunity to ease back into the routine gradually. My wrist is OK. I seem to be able to predict weather more than I used to, but I guess that comes with the territory. Hopefully, work will pick up in the spring.

Thanks to all, for your thoughts and prayers.

Earle & Judy

> Another glimmer of hope in the form of good news sparks this euphoric note from Judy. It is addressed to her supervisor at work. Her enthusiasm is unbridled and clearly obvious in the text of this personal note from her.
>
> Subsequent to the completion of the radiation, she also sends out the good news in a follow-up message to her friends and supporters. This joy, as we will soon see, was to be short-lived.

Wednesday, February 18, 2009

I'm so excited I [have] finally got some good news. My radiation doctor talked with me today. He is going to release me for work starting March 1st. I will finish my radiation the last Friday of February. He made me promise I wouldn't overdue it; don't push myself to work an eight hour day and make sure I continue to [keep] all my doctor appointments that I still have. It will take three to four weeks for the radiation tiredness to get through my body. My skin is really burned from the radiation. I can handle this!!!!!

I told Dr. K. that Wal-Mart is very good to me. They will not let me get overtired and do more than I should. After I sold myself, he finally agreed to let me return March 1st. I'm so excited.

I'm looking forward to returning to my team!!!

Have a great day, I am!!!!!

Judy

This is a personal message from Judy to her friends telling them of the latest development pertaining to her return to work. We have been pressing on under the impression that her return would be imminent. However, as new information became available to us, we learned differently.

This learning process was to become the norm rather than the exception as we traveled down this convoluted pathway we were on. Eventually, we came to expect as normal what we would have otherwise considered the abnormal.

This is a lesson that is not often mentioned in the official literature, but it is one which will stand anyone in a similar situation, in good stead.

Judy's Journey

Tuesday, February 24, 2009

I will NOT be returning to work on Monday. The doctor will not release me until my radiation burns are healed up. I am burned real badly on the chest, neck, underarm, and back. It is so bad in places, it is bubbled and oozing. I have three more days of radiation and they are hoping that I can get through them without having to give me a break. They check me over every day and the doctor will either say yes or no for the treatment.

I will let you know when they release me for work, but it does look like it will be a couple of weeks. Pray I can get through these next three days without taking a break; I really want to get this finished up.

Judy

Friday, February 27, 2009

I just wanted to let everyone know that I [am] finally finished with my radiation treatment. I'm severely burned and will take a few weeks to heal, but what a relief to have completed my 29 days.

Judy

So soon after the intense joy of the previous messages, we get the devastating news that there may be a serious problem. It is so critical in fact, that for the first time, the possibility of not returning to work is mentioned. To say this news was heartbreaking to Judy would be an enormous understatement. Devastating only begins to describe the effect of this newest development.

Monday, March 2, 2009

The first thing we have to report is that Judy's radiation treatments have been completed. It was a long haul and she has some nasty burns in the treated area. The doctor assures us, however, that with the application of the special ointment with which they supplied us, the burns will start to show significant improvement in the next couple of weeks. The healing can't come soon enough as far as I am concerned. Each time I apply the ointment, I feel so badly for Judy having to endure this.

Additional tests have also been completed. The results have confirmed that there is no heart damage from the administration of the Herceptin. Ongoing heart problems are one of the possible side effects of this drug, but the benefits far outweigh the potential side effects so the treatments will continue every three weeks until August.

The sad news is revealed by the PET scan. It indicates that the cancer appears to have spread to the lymph nodes in Judy's chest. The radiologist broke the news to us last Friday. The Oncology Center confirmed the report today.

At this time, we don't know what the treatment will be. We have been told that the radiation burns will have to be healed—to some extent at least—before starting any new treatment. I will report more on this as things develop.

The determination that the cancer has spread puts a new slant on Judy's status. Now, instead of her eagerly anticipated return to work, she will have to apply for long-term disability while her paperwork is being submitted to Social Security for Disability Retirement. She broke this news to her employer today. It was a sad day indeed. She loved her job and the folks she worked with. This is a tough turn of events for her to accept, but she is facing the challenge with the same determination and courage which has sustained her to this point.

We welcome and greatly appreciate all of your thoughts and prayers. We pray that we will be able to put this new situation and its far-reaching implications behind us soon. Thank you one and all for your concern.

Earle & Judy

This update opens with a faint hint of levity in a reference to the universally unpopular arrival and avoidance of Friday the 13th. This Friday the 13th would turn out to be a strangely ominous precursor of a decision to be made more than two years in the future. Though not particularly superstitious, I would choose to avoid that Friday the 13th too.

The information contained in the message did not reveal any new direction or momentous news. It simply outlines the recent progress and alludes to Judy's state of mind.

By this time, I had learned that the appetite for information and these updates was voracious. Because nearly two weeks had passed since the last installment, I had better get some news out to the hungry masses—or prepare to endure their wrath.

Saturday, March 14, 2009

I purposely chose to write this today rather than yesterday, which would have been Friday the 13th. Why chance it?

Today's report is not one of momentous news, but rather one of continued progress. Sometimes, the little steps forward are worth noting too.

First, Judy's radiation burns are healing. I was going to say "healing nicely," but the word nicely just does not seem applicable. The major affected region under her left arm has lost the red, raw look and has taken on the pinkish tint of any other healing burn. The remaining area in the lower quadrant of the treated site still has the look of an extremely sore burn. We are confident that with the continued use of the ointment, the inflammation will soon diminish as well. The remaining, less-affected areas are starting to look like healing sunburned patches, complete with the typical itchiness and flaking—a good sign indeed.

Judy's Journey

The other bit of progress is that we have an appointment for a consultation with the doctor who will be doing the surgical biopsy. This is an important step as it is essential to ascertain if the newly affected nodes are a spreading of the original cancer—a metastasis—or an outbreak of a new origin.

The results will determine which protocol they will use to fight it. While this is not a procedure we are looking forward to, it is definitely one that we are anxious to get beyond so that we can continue with the rest of the treatment.

Judy remains strong and is prepared to wage war and fight against this latest assault to her well-being. Knowing that she has the support of all of you is a tremendous boost to her spirits.

She is still incredibly saddened by having to give up her job. Because she will soon be busy combatting this newest development, we both recognize that she must marshal all of her reserves for the battle she now faces. The only apparent blessing here is that it may reduce the time she has to dwell on what she has had to forfeit to stay in the ring.

Again, thank you to everyone for your continued support, thoughts, and prayers. Know for a fact that they are all appreciated, and we are sure, a great help.

Earle & Judy

This update is somewhat more somber than most. In it, we outline what we know of the upcoming surgical biopsy. Because of the targeted locations' proximity to vital structures, some of the details are sobering.

Although not mentioned, this is dated two days before our 40th wedding anniversary—a time that should have been overflowing with joy and celebration. The upcoming occasion was, instead, filled with foreboding and uncertainty.

Friday, March 20, 2009

I should have sent this out yesterday, but by the time we returned home from two doctors' appointments (one for each of us) and a couple of errands, we were both exhausted. We came home and crashed.

We had the consultation with the surgeon who will be doing the surgical biopsy. He went into considerable detail about the procedure. The "details" were eye-opening to say the least. One of the target nodes is tucked up under the aorta which is a delicate place indeed. The other is somehow situated beneath the region where the blood vessels branch to go to the lungs. In order to perform the procedure, the surgeon will have to collapse one lung to enable him to safely access the area. As was the case in the previous biopsy, Judy will have to spend one night in the hospital to monitor her recovery. The surgeon, Dr. H., has come highly recommended. Everyone to whom we have spoken has confirmed that he is the absolute best in his field. Though it was for a less serious situation, he did a fine job the last time Judy required his surgical expertise; we fully expect he will do so again.

The oncologist wanted this done as soon as possible in order to ascertain what type of cancer with which he will be contending. The procedure is scheduled for Thursday the 26th.

In the interim, Judy is at a point in the process where she is feeling better than she has in weeks. The radiation-damaged areas have healed sufficiently that the affected vicinity is no longer an assortment of open sores. The side effects are diminished to the extent that she is able to taste and enjoy food again. Recently, since she is recuperating well from that phase and feeling more like herself, she has begun seeing friends and co-workers again. Before now, she hasn't really been up to much visiting. Her schedule has been busy to say the least, but she has truly enjoyed seeing as many folks as possible during this lull between treatments. The visits have been a source of encouragement and have helped her to replenish her resources.

We wish to thank each of you for your continued support and for keeping us in your thoughts and prayers. We are certain that all of this has helped us to this point and will continue to help us through the fight ahead.

Earle & Judy

The lead-in to this update should include fireworks, a marching band, and a fly-over. Simply saying "we have good news to report" is such a colossal understatement that I cannot imagine anything that would miss the mark by so much. The overwhelming joy reported here eclipses the feelings of uncertainty which permeated the previous message.

Included in the body of the text, we respectfully acknowledge the contribution of all of our supporters, thanking them once again. They have been praying for us—literally from all across the country. To be the recipients of such an outpouring of pure love and hope is indeed a humbling experience; also one for which we were truly grateful.

Thursday, March 26, 2009

I have so much to tell you that the thoughts are running through my head faster than I can sort them out. First, let me say that the biopsy results were better than anyone thought possible. Judy <u>does not</u> have cancer spreading to the lymph nodes as was suspected.

I must say that again—the biopsy came back showing NO CANCER—everything was **<u>benign</u>**.

I certainly understand if you have to go back over that again and let it sink in. We are still trying to fully grasp it ourselves. Let me try to tell you about this day.

We were to be at the Day Surgery area for 8:30 a.m. This meant an earlier wake-up call than what we have become accustomed to, but we made it there on time. The pre-op was as we have experienced in the past at the local hospital: thorough, professional, and friendly—oh, did I mention thorough? They ask so many questions, so many times to be certain of not only why you are there, but to be absolutely positive that you are, in fact, you. The process is so redundant it seems excessive, but we understand that it is to insure the patient's protection against undergoing an improper procedure. This is also where Judy's favorite part comes into play. Once they get you out of your clothes and into the hospital johnny, the nurse covers you over with a warm blanket. We tell them—only in jest, you understand—that if we didn't have to go through the surgery, we'd stop in once in a while just for the warm blanket.

The doctor was few minutes late. He had completed another surgery prior to Judy's. She tells me that when Dr. H. showed up, he was making humorous remarks just before entering the OR. This is very much *not* the serious surgeon whom we have known up until now. In the past, he has always been all business when we've met with him. It was nice to find out that he has a little sense of humor after all.

At 11:30 a.m., the surgeon came to the waiting room. He called me out into the hall and informed me of the good news. I was dumbstruck—literally speechless. He explained that the nodes in question were displaying signs of an infection—he had a Latin word for it which starts with an "S" and ends with an "—is." I couldn't be any more specific than that if my life depended on it.

The bottom line was: <u>the lymph nodes were not cancerous</u>!

Right here, I want to say to everyone who receives these updates (or reads them as "Forwards"): this is as much your victory as anyone's. If you are ever in a conversation when the power of prayer is questioned, feel free to recount this story. Tell them of the team of medical experts who sat on the "Tumor Board." All had agreed that the PET scan showed definite signs of the cancer having spread. Only a biopsy was needed to determine what type of cancer it was so they could decide which chemotherapy protocol was required to fight it. Be sure to tell them that the biopsy showed that, in fact, <u>no</u> cancer was present. If anyone should doubt your story, send them to me. I will tell them exactly what happened and how the collective prayers of many were answered on an otherwise ordinary day.

Coming just four days after our 40th Anniversary, we could not have asked for, or dreamed of receiving, a better gift. It was the gift of hope, renewal, and precious life itself.

The rest of the day unfolded as you might expect. Judy was transferred to a room (on the eighth floor) for post-op recovery. Since she was awake, alert, and in full control, naturally, she started right in issuing assignments and organizing life again! I was to do this, that, and the other thing. I had to call this one, that one, and the other one. I know when to ask questions and when to just do as I'm told—I left and followed orders. Early on in married life, I learned the absolute value of these two words: "Yes, dear."

When I returned, Judy was settled into her accommodations. Our daughter-in-law, Julie, was visiting. She was soon joined by other visitors: our daughter, Chris; a granddaughter; and a grandson. Later, my brother and his wife stopped in, as did another close friend. The nurses made several checks on Judy's recovery and declared that she was doing well. Just before we left, the surgeon, Dr. H., stopped in and reaffirmed that there was in fact, *no* cancer. After examining Judy, he confirmed that she had come through the operation with flying colors and was recovering nicely. He expects that she will be going home tomorrow morning.

I left her with the newspaper, the TV, a pile of scratch tickets, and most importantly, a smile. Judy's only complaint was that the IV was still in her arm.

As I have done in the past, I wish to thank each and every one of you for your continued support, prayers, and good thoughts. We now have proof of what wonderful things can happen when all that positive energy is focused and brought to bear against such an insidious beast as cancer. It also bears witness to the power of God.

From the bottom of my heart, thank you one and all. Thank you, thank you, and thank you.

Earle & Judy

This message is obviously a reply from Judy to her friend. It explains that she expects to be returning to work, but at a different assignment from that which she had been performing at the time she went out on disability. At this point, Judy had been having ongoing discussions with her supervisor at work. This was the option they agreed upon.

Saturday, March 28, 2009

Yes, but it will be doing a different job, still an office job. They have made up a job for me, it will be only part-time and I am working out the days and hours I want to work. I only want a job that I can work for two years because we have decided we are both retiring in two years. I need to get 15 years with Wal-Mart to keep certain benefits. July 8, 2011, will be 15 years.

They have been very good to me. They didn't have to find me an office job; they could have just thrown me out into the warehouse. We are very excited and hoping I can stay cancer-free, for a while anyway.

I am really tired today. I get very tired when I'm in the hospital. I didn't get released until 4:00 p.m., yesterday. Hope you are feeling better. I'll let you know when I'm supposed to return to work. I haven't been released yet. I don't see the doctor until April 8th.

Judy

This is another personal note from Judy to her boss at work. By this time, she has been completely out of work for about seven months. Her position at the company had to be filled. She accepted the fact that she would not be returning to the job she loved so much, even if the doctor released her. The management team had, however, created another position which was similar to her former job. They were presently holding it for her in anticipation of her return.

In typical Judy fashion, she expresses concern for her new boss being without his proper support staff while she is waiting to be declared fit for work. In spite of her circumstances and the personal impact, she still desires only the best for "her team" at Wal-Mart.

We also get a glimpse of the effect this is having on her morale. It is a reaffirmation of the determination that has carried Judy thus far in her courageous fight for life.

Saturday, April 4, 2009

[I] just returned from the doctor and hospital. It is 5:00 p.m. I'm thinking you have left for the day.

First of all, I'm really bumming right at this moment, but still have good spirits. I will beat all of this. They will not release me [to go] back to work yet and it will be at least May 4th, before I even can think about getting a work date. I went to the hospital for a chest X-ray this afternoon because of that cough and [the] pain I get in the chest area. I would have called you if I had gotten home sooner.

This infection that is growing in my chest is called zrotech (or something like that) and there are two kinds: a good kind and a bad kind. We are not sure what kind I have [see Sarcoidosis 4/8/09 update]. This could [have] developed from chemo, radiation, or just on its own. If it's the good kind, then it will clear up all by itself, if [the] bad kind, then it is treated with chemo, unless chemo created it, then it is treated with something else, but must get treated. It will attach to my lungs, if it has not already. You guessed it, going to a lung doctor on April 23rd for test[s]. The doctors will then decide what treatment, if any, I need. I will then see my cancer doctor on May 4th. They don't want to release me for work until they are completely confident that I'm healthy for work.

I was really looking forward to taking that position; I am and was very excited about working in dispatch for J. Please don't hold that job if J. needs to have his support person. I don't want to feel responsible for holding up the 6830 team for not having enough support. Please do what you have to do. I will just have to take each day and hope that you can take care of me if they release me.

I am bumming very much right now, tears just don't stop flowing, but I've been here before and things happen for a reason. Had a great visit with everyone today and miss all of you so much.

From the bottom to the top of my heart, I THANK ALL OF YOU for being so nice and supportive of me.

Your friend always,

Judy

Judy's Journey

Here, we outline the steps dictated by the new discovery which we were so pleased to recently report—because it was not cancer. This unexpected finding has created a new set of hurdles to overcome, but we are dealing with the situation. At this time, we are still blissfully unaware of the ominous shadow hanging over our heads. It has been roughly two weeks since we reported the tremendously good news following the biopsy. We are still floating on the euphoria of that development.

The information shared here, while disappointing, would pale by comparison to what would follow a mere month later. In retrospect, at this point, we had reached the zenith of our optimism throughout the entire process.

Wednesday, April 8, 2009

Judy had her appointment with the oncologist today. The news is somewhat mixed. He confirmed that the recent biopsy shows that the suspected nodes are not cancer. He explained that they have been affected by an infection which he referred to as "Sarcoidosis." He also explained that this infection can be serious in its own way.

Judy has to see a pulmonary specialist to assess the extent of the effect to her lungs. Her oncologist has declined to release her to go back to work until everything is identified and confirmed to be under control. While not the decision which she had desired, this seems to be the safe and sensible way to proceed at this time.

We are disappointed that the news is not the total clean slate that we had hoped for, but we are confident that the medical team is on top of the situation and we will come out OK in the end. We have learned to trust that her team has always had her best interests at heart.

As always, we thank you all for keeping us in your hearts and prayers. We are certain that they have all helped to get us to this point.

We hope you all have a Happy Easter and are able to enjoy it with your respective families and loved ones.

Earle & Judy

This update went out approximately one year into the "journey" as we had come to know it. Ironically, it was composed on a date that would prove to have an inexplicable habit of recurring as our story unfolded.

By this time, the recipients had become accustomed to receiving their updates from Judy—or me—depending upon whose contact list they were carried. The disclosure at the beginning of this message is to alert people that Judy is not currently managing her computer. I am the one who is presently attempting to perform the task of sending out the updates to both sets of contacts.

This message also contains the news which we had hoped never to have to deliver. It sets an entirely new tone for all messages which would follow.

Tuesday, May 5, 2009

Please note: although you are receiving this "from Judy," I (Earle), am the one sending it for her. She is not home to answer your replies, but if you wait a day or so she should be home and able to respond directly to you at that time.

Thanks.

E & J

I know that it has been a long time since the last update, but in my defense, not much was happening. Judy was regaining her strength and seemed to be progressing as expected. The main subject about which I was planning to report was the pulmonary test that she had last week. That has all changed due to some unforeseen developments.

Now, we have entered the next dreaded phase of the disease. The cancer has metastasized and spread to the brain. For the last two weeks, Judy has been experiencing a declining appetite and an onslaught of debilitating headaches. We were treating the headaches with Tylenol or Advil and it seemed to be helping. Then, this past Tuesday, I came home from work and found her curled up in a ball. I quickly learned that she had been sick to her stomach all day. She was unable to keep anything down, not even water. The doctor prescribed an anti-nausea medicine and instructed her to try to eat popsicles and drink water.

Her scheduled Herceptin treatment was set for Wednesday the 27th. She planned to speak to the oncologist about the situation then. He found her to be too dehydrated to have the treatment administered. An IV infusion was started to remediate the dehydration before attempting to start the Herceptin (which, you may recall, is the maintenance chemotherapy drug).

He also ordered an immediate MRI. The earliest appointment she could get was for 11:00 this morning. The doctor already had the results and was leaving a message on the answering machine ten minutes before she got home from the appointment. The MRI revealed evidence of the spread of the cancer to the brain.

Judy was to report to the Oncology Center at 2:30 p.m. for an initial treatment of a new medicinal cocktail—the name of which I couldn't repeat if I had to. The effect was that the headache started to dissipate within a few minutes of the IV.

The next step was to report directly to the hospital for inpatient admission. That is where she is now—in the hospital, on the sixth floor. She is not expected to be there much beyond tomorrow so visitors are not encouraged. For those who live in the area, her room phone number is (omitted). As we understand it, she will be going for her initial radiation appointment sometime tomorrow. If she is sufficiently hydrated and comfortable, she will be coming home tomorrow as well.

The radiation treatments will be administered to her as an outpatient. We don't have any specifics at this time as we have not spoken with the radiologist yet.

This has come as a complete shock to both of us. We always knew that this was a possibility, but we thought we had put the worst behind us for the immediate future. Now, we are not sure what to expect. Only one thing can be assured: we will face whatever develops with the same forthrightness that has been the lynchpin of our fight for the past year.

We hope you can find it in your heart and schedule to say a little prayer for Judy or keep her in your thoughts in some way. We feel strongly that it has been your combined prayers and thoughts which have helped to get Judy through the first stages of this battle.

We sure would appreciate them once again.

Thank you one and all.

Earle and Judy

> Now that the initial shock has passed, we are ready to settle in and fight this latest onslaught to Judy's well-being. We have to learn a new set of ground rules, but we are ready. We are eager to do whatever we must to regain what certainly seems like lost ground at this point.

Friday, May 29, 2009

I trust you have all heard the lyric "What a difference a day makes." Well, let me assure you we have just seen that "day"—twice in fact—and I can confirm the "What a difference" part from firsthand experience.

Just by happenstance, I had the day off today for a scheduled doctor's appointment (mine). Our plan was that I would check on Judy's progress through the night following my appointment.

Apparently, I was going up the visitor's elevator as she was going down on the staff side. When I reached her room, I was greeted by a partly eaten breakfast tray and a hospital employee who informed me that Judy had just left to go to radiology. Since that department is connected to the main hospital, I headed off immediately. I joined her there and we had our conference with the radiologist. Judy was then whisked off for her first treatment. They are not wasting any time with this treatment.

As the radiologist explained the plan to us, they will irradiate the entire brain during the first ten sessions. In the last four, they will concentrate on the four spots that lit up in the MRI. The objective of the first round of protocol treatments is, hopefully, to destroy any undetected cells that may have escaped detection and had somehow not been revealed by the MRI. The second series of concentrated treatments are intended to ensure maximum exposure in the heavily-affected, identified areas.

He further explained that the brain does not respond well to chemotherapy due to the manner in which human physiology is structured, intending to provide maximum protection to the brain. Without getting too technical, something called the "Blood-Brain Barrier" prevents large molecules—both good and bad ones—from invading the brain. Unfortunately, this same protective mechanism also blocks large molecular medicinal compounds as well. It keeps them from reaching the brain to effectively target infections, tumors, etc. This explains more clearly why the ongoing Herceptin treatments—which are supposed to protect against further development of the cancer throughout the body—do not protect the brain. This also explains why the brain is the most common spot that a cancer targets when it redevelops. Obviously, this has not caught the doctors unprepared. They have a plan and they are confident that this can be controlled.

Back to the "day":
All of this took up most of the morning. We were back to her room by about 11:00 a.m. or so, just in time for her "hospitalist"—I swear that is his title—Dr. F. to stop by, ask a few questions, complete his examination, and offer to discharge her. Of course, we readily accepted the offer and we were headed home by 12:30 p.m.

Judy is home now. She feels better. The meds have resolved the headache and she is able to keep some food down. We stopped for a coffee frappe on the way home. The serving size that used to last most of an afternoon was gone before we were even halfway home.

We are confident in the doctors' ability to lead us through this maze. We are settled in for this fight. We remain completely committed to each other.

We are fully aware and appreciative of everything that all of you have done, and are doing, to help us in this battle. We are grateful for all your thoughts and prayers. We are sure that it is the combined efforts of all of you, as well as those of the medical community, which have brought us to this point and will see us through this latest challenge.

Thank you one and all.

Earle and Judy

> Here is one of the numerous personal messages that Judy sent to her friends and supporters addressing one of the many logistical transportation challenges. This one concerns an eye appointment. Judy not only arranged a ride to an appointment this way, but as was typical of her way of multi-tasking, she also managed to combine the transportation request with a social visit. These serendipitous outings provided priceless encouragement. They served to keep Judy's spirits high and boost her morale.

Monday, June 1, 2009

My eye appointment is not until July 27th at 1:00 p.m. I would still like you to take me even though I can drive [right now], but they will dilate my eyes and I [will] have a hard time driving then. Maybe you can come down early and we can do lunch or something. Let me know.

Judy

> Now the brain treatment protocol has begun in earnest. The radiation is administered every day. This has created a huge transportation stumbling block. Because I am still working at this time, the majority of the shuttling to and from the center has fallen to the stalwart group of friends and family who have volunteered to help out.

> These opportune visits were so welcomed and very much appreciated by Judy. Unfortunately, I have had to forewarn all who step in to help that they need to be prepared to deal with the unpredictable changes in Judy's condition. Newly developing circumstances create fluctuating degrees of stamina and strength. Other developments initiate varying challenges that now impact Judy on a daily basis.

> In spite of these ordeals, somehow, we managed to proceed—one day at a time.

Saturday, June 6, 2009

It seems that we have entered the "new things every day zone" with Judy's situation.

The first full week of radiation treatment is now behind us. From what we can tell, it would seem to have gone as well as can reasonably be expected. A special thanks to everyone who volunteered and provided transportation as well as emotional support.

The latest development comes from our primary care physician, Dr. T. He had scheduled a rather extensive appointment with Judy this week. He is following up on things which are not part of the specific focus of the oncologist or the radiologist because they are not directly related to the cancer. Her PCP is concerned about Judy's overall health and well-being. He is addressing the shortness of breath and possible heart issues which seem to be a result of the chemo. He has ordered some tests this week to establish baselines for purposes of comparison. These results will enable him to judge her progress. Though this has added to the daily regimen of hospital visits, we accept that they are necessary. We are also glad that she has so many healthcare providers in her court.

A special note here to everyone who has so graciously volunteered to help with transportation. First, our heartfelt thanks for what you are doing. Not only have you resolved the ride issue, but Judy gets a great deal of pleasure out of seeing all of you.

For future providers, there is another thing you need to be aware of: due to the pressure of one of the tumors in the back of her head, Judy is becoming less stable on her feet. It is not a critical issue yet, but it would be best if someone walks at her side when she goes in for the treatments—just as a precaution.

As always, we wish to thank each and every one of you for your good thoughts, prayers, and positive support.

We continue to believe they help. Thank you one and all.

Earle and Judy

> Judy and her boss would frequently speak on the phone. It would seem that this message to her supervisor probably followed a telephone conversation they must have had earlier.
>
> Judy was highly pragmatic concerning her situation. On occasion, the people with whom she spoke were less than eager to confront the reality of her condition.
>
> I suppose human nature is often in denial, particularly when it comes to dealing with potentially terminal conditions. In retrospect, I suspect this message was meant to counter one of those calls.

Tuesday, June 9, 2009

I didn't mean to upset you today, but you must understand the reality of my situation. I feel privileged to have worked for you and to know you as a great friend. We have had an enjoyable time chatting and sharing stories of our families.

I will be around for a while. The doctors still have a few things up their sleeve. As long as my body responds to the treatment, I will be here. Thanks.

I feel privileged knowing you and your family and you do have a wonderful family.

Please say hello to C for me.

Judy

This rather lengthy update was written in two sessions over the course of the entire day. The uncertainty of the treatments and the new side effects are discussed. Also, what would prove to be one of the most intense phases in the course of treatment is hinted at.

At the time of this update, Judy is maintaining her stalwart composure, but cracks are beginning to show. The physical toll is becoming more apparent.

An important trip to visit an uncle is mentioned here as well. This trip had been planned for the preceding year, but had to be postponed due to the intense treatment schedule at that time. The anticipated excursion meant a lot to Judy and was one of those goals that she had set for herself. Setting these objectives gave her something positive to focus upon. They also represented rewards for following the doctor's orders and managing to get through the current medical protocol.

Friday, June 12, 2009

This week has been another roller coaster ride. On Tuesday, the doctor suspected that the medications were not working as expected since the pressure was not going down quickly enough. For the first time, surgery was discussed and Dr. J. was called in. As you can imagine, this was disturbing news for us. The one positive aspect is that we know Dr. J. from our previous, firsthand interactions. He was the neurosurgeon who successfully removed Judy's benign brain tumor six years ago. He is a very good surgeon and is well-respected in his field.

On Wednesday, it was determined that the medications were in fact working and surgery would not be needed. What a relief that was for both of us. Judy continues to experience residual treatment side effects. Her balance is still affected and her memory isn't as sharp as before the treatments.

On Tuesday, her speech seemed to be impacted, but now, since the pressure has been reduced, that seems to have improved. She continues to require more than her usual amount of rest, but her body is being taxed on many fronts. That was one of the things the radiologist advised us would likely happen.

Today, it is my turn to take her to the treatment appointment. I am hoping to have a chance to meet with Dr. K. and get some firsthand information on her progress. I'll pass along whatever news he may have.

(Later in the day)
Today's visit went well. The doctor is pleased with the way the treatment is progressing. He reduced the steroids by 25% for the weekend. If she tolerates this well, on Monday he wants to try to drop them again by the same amount. We have been charged with the

responsibility of remaining alert for the symptoms: primarily, headaches and/or speech and balance impairments which hopefully, don't return.

He further outlined the treatment plan. The final, whole-brain radiation will be delivered this Thursday. Following that, they want to wait three to four weeks to schedule a new MRI. Once they can compare that to the original, they can draw up the treatment plan for the next phase.

Compared to last Tuesday, Judy is much better. She continues to run out of steam quickly. This becomes even more noticeable when she misses a nap.

The doctor gave his approval for the trip which we have planned over the 4th of July holiday. Judy is pleased and is doing all she can to ensure that we will be able to visit her uncle in North Carolina as we had originally planned to do last year.

Thanks again to all of you for the good thoughts and prayers. A special thanks once again to everyone who has volunteered to provide transportation during the radiation treatments. We couldn't have made it through this without your help.

Thank you one and all.

Earle and Judy

Judy's Journey

Now, the dreaded roller coaster is headed on that downward spiral again; this time with confirmation of our worst fears. As if the type of breast cancer (IBC) Judy battles wasn't bad enough, here, we learn that the particular type of brain cancer that she has developed is equally dreaded, and possibly worse.

Devastating only hints at how this latest news crashes into our lives. Here, once again, Judy's strength and perseverance come to the forefront as we share this latest development with our news-hungry supporters.

Friday, June 19, 2009

It's going to take some 'doing' to get through this update, please bear with me if it takes some time to finish.

On Wednesday the 17th, Judy had a Herceptin treatment and met with Dr. B., the oncologist. He explained that the difficulties she is experiencing are due to the unavoidable combination of the steroids and the radiation. Her skin is so tender; the slightest touch leaves a nasty-looking bruise. It's surprising how many times you can bump a leg or an arm and do not even realize it under ordinary conditions.

Currently, Judy is at the lowest level of endurance she has experienced throughout this entire battle. The oncologist assured her that as soon as the radiation is over and we are able to wean her off the steroids her stamina will return fairly rapidly. This is good news at a time when good news is in short supply.

He further explained that the form of brain cancer which has developed is one of, if not the, worst types known. What they do know is that the cancer is not curable. That is not to say that it can't be treated; it definitely can, but at this time there is no known cancer protocol that will eradicate it completely. He has assured us that the treatments currently available will enable her to enjoy a period of what they refer to as "quality life."

Needless to say, the last few days here have been filled with every emotion imaginable; everything from rage to incredulous disbelief. Regardless of the medical pronouncements, Judy and I have determined to put all that behind us and face this latest development head-on. We accept that whatever happens is part of a greater plan that we do not—and cannot—understand. We recognize that we must accept it. We will deal with it as we have everything else to this point—together. We will continue to follow the recommendations of the medical team which has brought us to this point. There remains a possibility of surgery in the future and there are also treatments on the horizon that may be of value—if and when they become available. We will continue to keep everyone informed through these updates when there is significant news to relay.

In our plan, I will continue to work toward my anticipated retirement in about a year and a half. This will keep our health insurance in force and put me at the magic age of 62 when I retire. That will allow me to take advantage of the best retirement benefits, with insurance, in the quickest time frame possible. Beyond that, we plan to do whatever Judy's condition will allow.

Judy's Journey

As ever, thanks to everyone for keeping us in your thoughts and prayers. We cannot adequately describe how much this means to us.

Thank you one and all.

Earle and Judy

> By now, we should have been ready for and expecting the unexpected, but the news in these next two updates took everyone by complete surprise. The first note went out very late at night and only touches on the events of the day.
>
> The message which follows goes into more detail about an experience that will profoundly influence every decision in our lives from this day forward. It was this single event that finally prodded me into getting the much-hated and long-resisted cell phone. I would never again allow myself to be "unreachable" at work.

Tuesday, June 23, 2009

This is going to be the shortest update ever. I'll try to send out the full story tomorrow. It is just too late tonight for more than the abbreviated version.

This morning, Judy was rushed to the ER with severe abdominal pains. An MRI determined that she had a perforated bowel and emergency surgery was needed. She has already had the surgery. She was out of the recovery room and had been transferred to a regular room when I left the hospital at about 9:00 p.m. She was still very groggy, but the doctor assured us that she will be fine.

Recovery is expected to be a lengthy process. All travel plans for the summer are currently on hold. I'll fill in the gaps tomorrow and answer questions should any arise.

Thanks for keeping us in your hearts and thoughts.

Earle and Judy

Wednesday, June 24, 2009

A full day has passed. Things are beginning to look a little brighter after 24 hours. Though still very serious, Judy has a long road to recovery, but everything seems to be more attainable today.

Now, for the detailed report that I promised you last night ...

Yesterday at about 8:00 a.m., Judy was suddenly struck with sharp, shooting, stabbing pains in her abdomen. At first, she was unsure what to do, but when they persisted, she called our daughter, Christina, to have her contact the doctor for his opinion. Once he was reached and understood the situation, he advised them to get her to the Emergency Room ASAP.

I was at work and Chris was tied up with extra kids. Enter our "on-call angel," E. She dropped everything and rushed Judy to the ER. I immediately arranged to get out of work and met them at the hospital shortly after they arrived there. At that time, we did not have a clear understanding of the urgency of the situation. We expected them to schedule an MRI and admit her to a room for observation.

Judy and I decided that while that was going on, I would get her car serviced in order for it to be ready for our upcoming trip to North Carolina next week. If this seems nonchalant, I must reiterate: at the time, neither of us had any idea how serious the condition was. We both expected some tests, medical exams, and lots of waiting before an eventual discharge home. Because the trip—which meant so much to Judy—was imminent, it made sense to both of us that I should try to accomplish something constructive; rather than just stand by waiting for test results.

When I returned, I fully expected Judy to have been admitted to a room, so I inquired at the front desk. When I was directed to the second floor surgical waiting room, I was confused, disturbed, and more than a little apprehensive, to say the least. I went straight to the Day Surgery admitting area and—as calmly as I could manage—demanded some information. I got just enough of a briefing to understand that something critical was unfolding and accepted my role as the waiting relative. Later, a nurse came out and filled in most of the blanks.

The MRI results showed evidence of a ruptured intestine, but the debris was so extensive that they could not determine the exact location of the breach. Emergency surgery was required to visualize, assess, and clean the area sufficiently to permit the surgeon to locate the point of perforation, decide the best approach to affect a repair, quickly accomplish the task at hand and in a nutshell—save Judy's life.

The surgery lasted about an hour and a half. The recovery room stay was another hour. Following the completion of the surgery, the doctor explained in some detail what had happened and why. It was evidently the result of a combination of things. This life-threatening incident had been, in part, an adverse event resulting from the medication treatment—the steroids—complicated by Judy's weakened state of health as her body waged its fight against the invading cancer. In Judy's case, the treatment was at least as bad as the disease she had been battling for more than a year. At this point, it was quite possibly even harsher. It certainly struck with more immediate potential lethality.

Last night, Judy was still very much under the influence of the anesthesia and certainly less than 100% coherent. This afternoon when I visited, she was much more awake, alert, and aware of the situation. She is, of course, disappointed that this monkey wrench will cancel our summer plans, at least for the time being. She fully understands the severity and seriousness of what has happened. She has vowed to fight this as hard as she has been battling the cancer. She stated that her goal now is to recover sufficiently to participate in the scheduled *Walk for Breast Cancer* fund raiser in Manchester this October. Knowing Judy as I do, I have no doubt that she will be there.

Judy's Journey

The doctor has told us to anticipate that Judy will be in the hospital until early next week. She is then expected to spend a month or so in a rehabilitation facility. This will allow her the opportunity to heal, regain her strength, and work with therapists to get back on her feet. She must get her body back to a state of health sufficient to allow the surgeon to operate once more to complete the needed repairs to her intestinal system. We are told to expect this part of the recovery phase to last a minimum of four months, but it could take longer.

In the meantime, Judy has recovered enough that I came home from today's visit with a "to-do" list that covered the back of a 6x9 envelope. Some things never change! She is in good spirits, comfortable, and experiencing only a minimum amount of pain.

For anyone in the area, she is at the hospital in Manchester. When I left tonight, she was in Room (omitted). There was talk of moving her to another room; she will still be on the eighth floor though. She is able to have visitors, but I would caution anyone going in to be alert for signs of fatigue and not stay too long. Also, do not take her any food as she is not allowed to eat solids at this time. Judy has obviously been through a lot and rest is the vital element necessary to promote healing, in fact, it is the top priority for her recovery.

As always, we extend our heartfelt thanks to everyone for keeping us in your thoughts and prayers. We are sincerely grateful to you all.

Earle and Judy

This short note went out from me via Judy's computer to advise the folks on her contact list that the updates they were about to receive were not actually from Judy. I was serving as a substitute version of Judy, communicating directly from her laptop.

My ultimate plan was to avoid a flood of replies from people expecting to hear back from Judy. I was only partially successful.

Wednesday, June 24, 2009

This is really Earle here, not Judy. I am letting everyone know that it will be several days before Judy will be able to use her computer. Please refrain from sending her new mail until Judy informs you that she is back on line.

I will continue to send out the updates from her computer as they come up.

Thank you.

Earle

As reported here, Judy's rebound following the unexpected emergency surgery was amazing. This, no doubt, was largely due to her positive approach to everything that this dreadful malady, as well as its treatment and complications, had thrown at her. We also give a great deal of credit to the legions of supporters who were following her every move.

Judy's Journey

As outlined in this message, Judy would be relocating to a Rehab facility soon. We were excited about the move because it was a hallmark of improvement.

Unfortunately, as we had experienced time and time again in the roller coaster ride of *Judy's Journey*, this was an emotion that would soon reverse itself once again.

Friday, June 26, 2009

There were major developments today. The doctor has determined that Judy's post-op progress is some two days ahead of schedule or at least ahead of what they had expected. This improvement has been evidenced by the fact that she went from a first "meal" of tea, broth, and Jell-O Thursday evening, to meals very close to normal today. Friday brought macaroni and cheese, a tuna sandwich, and clam chowder. These culinary accomplishments and the removal of all tubes and medical connections have led to the next big step.

Tomorrow morning (Saturday), Judy will be discharged from the hospital and transferred to a medical rehab unit. She will be going to a facility located close to home. We are familiar with this establishment; historically, we knew it to be a good facility. The original plan proposed that she would spend approximately one month in rehabilitation. The doctor has indicated that if her progress continues at the present pace, it is possible that the rehab stay could be shorter.

Good news indeed.

Today was the last day of the steroid weaning program. Judy is now completely off the troublesome drug that was such a beneficial part of the treatment program— and conversely, also created such a deadly threat. More good news: the doctor says that the lingering side effects of the steroids should be significantly reduced in a week or so. From this point forward, we would be ever-vigilant whenever any of Judy's healthcare providers even hinted at initiating steroids again.

While at rehab, she will be working on all forms of rehabilitation therapy designed to get her back on her feet and headed home. We don't yet know any details of what the schedule will be while she is there. When we have more information, we will pass it along. For now, we are pleased with the progress she has made. We look forward to continued improvement and Judy's eventual return home.

As always, we wish to thank you all for keeping us in your thoughts and prayers. There can be no doubt that they have helped us to reach this milestone in Judy's recovery.

Earle and Judy

Saturday, June 27, 2009

This will be a quick note to let everyone know that Judy made the move to the rehab facility today. What was billed as a "first thing this morning" event finally occurred this afternoon about 2:30 p.m. This created a long day for everybody. Judy has already started walking a little more and is unwavering in her determination to work hard and improve sufficiently to return home.

It helped her mood a little when I was able to locate the Red Sox game on her TV this afternoon. There is no printed guide for the stations so it took a little searching, but we found them—even better, they won 1-0!

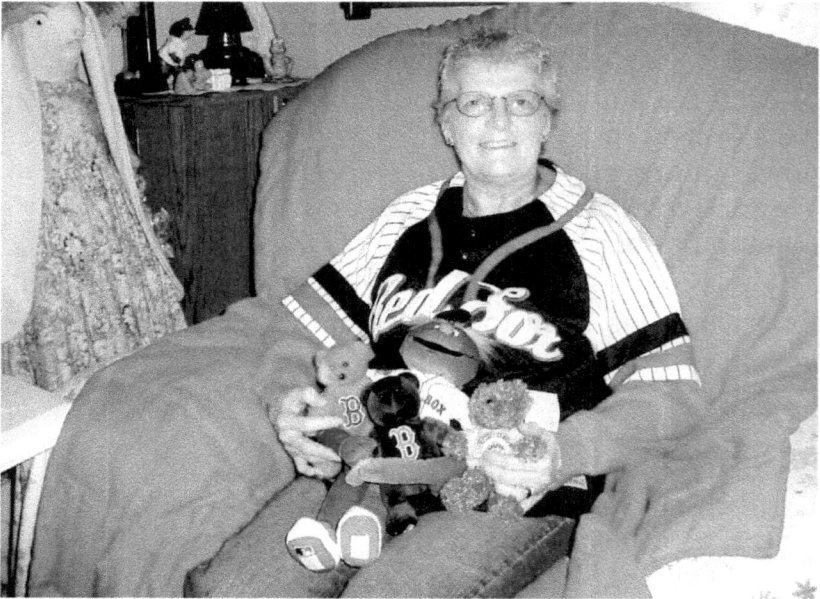

Judy, the ever-devoted Boston Red Sox fan!

She was told to expect therapy sessions seven days a week. I'm not sure if that will be the case or not. Guess we'll find out tomorrow. She is unwavering in her intent to work hard and meet whatever goals they set in order to shorten her stay there.

Special note to those in the immediate area; Judy is more than somewhat apprehensive regarding this move. If any of you are able to find time in your schedule to stop by for a quick visit or possibly a call, she is at the (name omitted) Rehabilitation Center. She is in Room (omitted) and her direct phone number is (omitted). She could definitely use a little cheering up and encouragement right now. Should anyone care to send a card to the house, I pick up the mail daily and will take whatever comes in for her directly to her.

Thanks to you all for your most generous support.

Earle

> Here is the report on the first full day at the rehabilitation center. At this point, we still have a high degree of confidence in the facility and the staff there. This opinion of their skills is to be short-lived.

Sunday, June 28, 2009

Judy has now spent a full day in the rehab facility. There are some small hurdles to surmount, but most were probably the result of coming onboard during the weekend when the full-time staff was off. We do know the answer to "Will there be physical therapy on Sunday?" The answer is "Yes." I was there when the therapist came in to take her for her physical therapy session.

Her day went well. She had enough company to keep her sufficiently distracted. She also admitted to me that the food here was good. We watched the Red Sox game, a disappointing loss, but nevertheless a great game to watch. She has her own wardrobe and is much more comfortable wearing her own clothes again.

Her spirits seem to have returned to normal levels. She is determined to work hard at the therapies and minimize her stay as much as possible. She is already doing more than she has been able to do for the past week. The steroids are working their way out of her system and the ill effects are diminishing.

Unfortunately, the beneficial effects that they were producing are decreasing as well. Some of the previous negative side effects of the chemotherapy, particularly the pain in her feet, which had been reduced—or masked—by the steroids, are returning. This is a disturbing turn of events, but one with which she has dealt before so we don't expect it to slow her down.

I'll know more tomorrow when I get a report on what happens on a weekday. I will let you know how that goes in the next update. For now, I am just happy to report that she is back to making progress and she has a more positive outlook.

Thanks to all for keeping us in your hearts.

Earle

At this point we have spent a full weekday in the rehab unit and we are working out the small details that can be so annoying. The progress seems to be advancing at a brisk rate.

A target date, or time frame for discharge, has already been discussed. Without question, the main goal of her care planning is Judy's return home. It is the number one priority for both of us at this juncture in the program.

Monday, June 29, 2009

Today's visit with Judy was encouraging. She has met most of the regular staff; she is in good spirits; and she has a goal. They told her that the plan is to get her well enough to go home in two weeks. If I understood correctly, the evaluation of the week's progress is normally scheduled for Thursdays.

Judy is doing more and more for herself now, getting dressed, etc., and is improving daily. Her feet are still a problem, but they are dealing with it. The PT is going well. They have identified that one leg does not have the same level of strength as the other. At this point, the focus of their efforts is to concentrate on equalizing bilateral strength.

I have solved the problem of the inadequate TV remote. The unit that came with the room would only allow her to change the channel by using the "up" arrow or the "down" arrow. This presents a problem when you wish to change from channel 4 to channel 51 (where the Red

Sox games are). I picked up a universal remote with a number pad and set it up to control the TV in the room. There is now one less frustration for her to deal with.

She is doing well; in fact, well enough that I again heard those three words that I had gotten so used to hearing when I'd come home from work: "I've been thinking ..." This is usually followed by a project or task of some sort. I hadn't heard that infamous declaration for at least a week. This is a clear indication to me that she is getting better.

As always, we send our thanks to everyone for keeping us in your thoughts and prayers.

Thank you.

Earle and Judy

Judy has been in rehab for about a week and a half now and much has happened during that time. In spite of the incident mentioned here, which will forever taint our opinion of the facility, Judy has been making progress and will soon be returning home.

The outcome of the emergency surgery to repair the colon rupture was, what was expected to be, a temporary colostomy. One of the goals of rehab has been the fitting of a colostomy system and mastering the challenges of self-care techniques that would be required until she had achieved sufficient healing for it to be reversed. Initially, this was a source of much sensitivity for Judy. Although it would become an essential part of all our logistical planning in the future, this, like so many other unexpected adaptations, was soon taken in stride—and simply dealt with.

Wednesday, July 8, 2009

I know it has been a while since my last update. I have been waiting for something of note to report rather than simply rehashing the day's events. Well, all good things come to he who waits; patience is a virtue; and whatever other tried and true expressions you can think of. The waiting has paid off. We were expecting to schedule a Thursday evaluation and we have been informed instead that, barring any unforeseen event between now and Saturday the 11th, they intend to discharge Judy home this Saturday.

We aren't certain, but we think that this sudden push to discharge Judy is, at least somewhat, connected to an incident that occurred a few days ago. What incident you say? When they dropped her! The therapist was having her walk up a set of practice stairs and was not beside her while the exercise was being performed. Judy had clearly informed them that her right leg was not strong, but the "know-it-all" therapist paid no heed to her statement. As a consequence, Judy collapsed on the stairs with no one at her side for assistance. It goes without saying, the attitude of everyone in the facility changed dramatically following that event. We believe that this unexpected decision to send her home a bit prematurely is, at least in some way, related to their newly realized vulnerability. At this juncture, we don't care why. We are just happy to be going home.

Judy's Journey

Judy will have a visiting nurse stop in once a day, and we think there may be home-based PT sessions as well, but the "take-home message" is that she will be HOME!! It looks like my bachelor days are numbered. The fish will be thrilled to have her home so they can be properly fed once again. I'll just be glad to have her home.

We knew she was making good progress, but I don't think we realized how much she had advanced. Her PT today and during the next few days will focus on improving her walking and stair-climbing skills. She reports that the workouts have become more intense lately. I guess that is for the big push to make the stated goal of an early discharge.

I simply cannot convey how much the possibility of an early discharge means to us. I can, however, say that we sincerely appreciate all of your support, prayers, and good thoughts. As always, they have helped provide the strength, direction, and endurance to reach this important milestone.

Thank you one and all.

Earle & Judy

We are getting closer to the planned discharge date. All of the loose ends seem to be coming together simultaneously as evidenced in this update. The intensity of the therapy is picking up and my home preparation assignments are falling in line.

We are increasingly certain that we will be able to meet the Saturday goal, but we are hesitant to take our eye off the mark lest some unexpected glitch crop up to foil our departure objectives.   For both of us, the anticipation of Judy's homecoming is palpable.

Thursday, July 9, 2009

This will be just a quick note to keep everyone up-to-date. The plan is still to have Judy home this Saturday.

She achieved two major milestones today. To say we are excited about them is a profound understatement. This morning she was "taught" how to take a shower. Amazing to think that you would have to be taught something as mundane as daily hygiene techniques, but Judy has many additional issues which must be taken into consideration now. These concerns add another whole dimension to a variety of otherwise commonplace tasks. The teaching method was "by doing" so she had the opportunity to experience her first real shower since this latest episode began. That started her day on an unparalleled high note. She was still talking about it when I visited after lunch.

Her afternoon therapy session was focused on stair climbing. It included a climb up; a return, going part of the way down and back up again; and finally completing the downward progression on a set of practice steps.   This was a major hurdle to have surmounted. Just a few days ago, this was the task she was attempting when she collapsed.   Today, the endeavor was 100% successful. She was so elated that she called me as soon as she got back to her room. These accomplishments bode well for her return home in just two days.

I was busy today playing the part of coordinator—a hat that Judy wears much better than I. My "Honey Do" list included arranging for, and picking up various items and supplies that we will need when she comes home. What I don't yet have in place will be delivered tomorrow morning. Don't you just love it when a plan comes together with relative ease?

Judy's improvement over the past two or three days has been amazing. Of course, she deserves the lion's share of the credit for her tenacity, determination, and the will to beat this.

At this time, we are in all of your debt for your strong support, good thoughts, and prayers. Know in your hearts that we thank you, one and all.

Earle and Judy

> The much-anticipated day has finally arrived and everything has gone well. This quick note went out to assure our supporters that we had met the planned deadline and that we were, in fact, home.

Saturday, July 11, 2009

The message will be short and sweet today. We—and by we, I mean Judy and I—are HOME. I went in to pick her up about 7:30 this morning. She was just finishing up with the final nurse-related procedures. I packed up what was left in her wardrobe, walked her out to the car, and we headed off to Moe Joe's for a breakfast celebration.

We arrived home about 9:30 a.m. and Judy was able to negotiate her way into and around the house. She is presently "at home" in her favorite chair and going through her e-mails. She has indicated that she intends to send out a personal message later when she has caught her breath and settled in (that may mean after a nap—I'm not sure). As for now, she is in good spirits. She is a lot stronger than I expected her to be and just glad to be home.

Thanks to all for your continued support.

Earle & Judy

This particular Saturday was a busy day to say the least. In addition to the customary update that I sent out, Judy sent these next two messages personally.

The first was to her general contact list. Judy was always one to express appreciation; she takes this opportunity to thank them all for their support.

The second was to her boss at work informing him of her planned participation in an upcoming fundraising walk which was being arranged by an acquaintance via a shop in town. The event was entitled "Jump for Judy" but was actually promoting two individuals who were battling breast cancer—both were named Judy. Below,

I have also included the message to which Judy refers in her note.

Saturday, July 11, 2009

THANK YOU! Earle and I wish to say **THANK YOU** to everyone for all the flowers, gifts, visits, phone calls, support, and all the prayers for me during this latest episode.

It's your support that helps keep my spirits up. I know I can depend on any of you when needed. My goal is to be walking and driving in the next couple of weeks. Earle is my ANGEL and I couldn't have gotten this far without him.

THANK YOU FOR EVERYTHING!!

Love

Earle & Judy

Saturday, July 11, 2009

(To her boss)
This is the site I was telling you about. "Jump for Judy" is where donations are made or if you want to walk with me. *"The Sampler"* is the shop that Barbara owns.

Make sure you use my name when you go there ... Miss
you and I feel great today.

LoL (Lots of Love)

Judy

(Below is the notice to which Judy referred in the above
message.)

From: Barbara
Subject: Please walk with me

*I wanted to let you know how much you
inspire me and I hope you'll join me in
inspiring others.   Since you have been
touched by breast cancer firsthand, I would
be honored if you would join me at the
<u>American Cancer Society Making Strides
Against Breast Cancer Walk</u>.*

*As a breast cancer survivor, you're part of a
group of more than 11 million people across
the country which has battled cancer and
won. You're also part of an even larger
community of caring people who support the
ongoing fight against breast cancer.*

*Every year, <u>Making Strides</u> brings together
people with a never-ending passion to fight
breast cancer for an inspiring day of
friendship, remembrance, and hope. It's an*

Judy's Journey

incredible day–one I'm truly looking forward to–and I hope you will join me.

After a week at home and adjusting to the new routine, this optimistic update is a welcome accounting of the past few days' activities. Judy continues to show progress. We are adapting to the rigors of what will prove to be the new normal in our lives—incorporating the recently added personal care element—addressing the daily requirements of living with a colostomy.

Although it was rarely mentioned either in updates or conversation, the logistics of dealing with this new system would be at the forefront of all arrangements and future plans. It would have a direct bearing on every decision we made, especially concerning outings; everything from going out to dinner, to whether or not we would be able to complete any of our future travel plans. It is easy to underestimate the far-reaching effects that this procedure can have on someone's life. Eventually, Judy took it in stride just as she had done with every other hurdle she had encountered and would face in the future. Her strength and determination was an inspiration to me and to all who knew her.

Sunday, July 19, 2009

Yesterday marked one week home for Judy. She has continued to show improvement on a daily basis. Each day brings small increments of recovery in her fight to return to some sort of normalcy. Since returning home, she has all but given up the need to use the walker; she is able to manage stairs with supervision; and she has mastered getting in and out of the car on her own. While to many, these may seem like extremely small strides, what really counts is that they are progressive steps moving in the right direction.

Today's highlight was the first real shower at home. This was a huge step and definitely a much-welcomed one for Judy. She still gets tired easily, but is improving in that respect as well.

The biggest obstacle that she still has to overcome is her lack of appetite. This is a problem which we believe is a residual effect of the radiation. We are hopeful that it will continue to improve in time. In the interim, we are assuring that she is getting adequate nutrition by way of *Ensure* supplements and fortified instant breakfast drinks. The one thing that she seems to be able to get down is hot cereal like oatmeal and cream of wheat. I am guessing that when this is over she'll never want either again.

We have settled into the home-care routine. I am honing my "nursing" skills and Judy is showing great potential as an ideal patient. I am on vacation and will be able to take Judy to her multiple appointments this week. The first appointment is with the surgeon. We are hoping that the staples will be coming out at that time. Should that be the case, it will dramatically decrease my nursing duties as changing the dressings have been a big part of my responsibilities.

As always, we want to thank each of you for your continued support and for keeping us in your hearts and prayers. Once again, Judy is on the mend and we are certain that we are at this point due, in no small part, to your encouragement and support. Thank you one and all.

Earle & Judy

> Here, we read a short note from Judy to her friend Lynda explaining why she will not need the ride to an appointment which they had arranged earlier.
>
> Reference is also made to a difficulty in walking. This would remain a troublesome problem for some time. Through it all, Judy still maintains that she is "doing OK."

Friday, July 24, 2009

Thank you for my birthday card. Also, Earle will be taking me to my eye appointment on Monday. He is still on vacation and he wants to be there for the visit. My vision is getting blurry from the radiation, which we knew could happen. If I have any follow-ups, I will let you know if I need a ride.

I'm doing OK. [I] still hate the taste of food. The doctor says to be patient and the taste buds will come back in time, but it will take time.

I am walking better. I still have trouble with the right leg from the fall at rehab. I [will] have X-rays and ultrasound done on it today. They are looking to see if anything is going on with it. It feels like an elephant leg all the time, very heavy.

Well, I'm tired. We had three appointments today—none of them short. I will chat with you later.

Don't work too hard.

Judy

> Now, approximately two weeks have passed. Apparently the clamor from the update recipients has filtered back to me, clearly making the point that there had been a lack of news. The universal question was "What has been happening and why haven't we heard anything?" When this would occur I would again try to assuage their anxiety with the "no news is good news" idiom—a tactic that never really worked.
>
> In this update, I had to resort to recounting Judy's new diet and her adventures on the deck to fill the space. Such was the hunger for reports from her supporters that any news was welcome.

Saturday, August 8, 2009

It has occurred to me, or I should say it has been pointed out to me, that it has been a while since the last update and it is time for one. In my defense, let me remind you all again that in this case, the "no news is good news" guideline applies.

Judy's Journey

Since the last time we were in contact, Judy has continued to make progress. To be sure, the improvement has been in small increments, but every bit of forward movement is welcome.

She is walking much better. Her confidence level has improved greatly and I have observed her progress in negotiating the stairs. She still only tackles stairs with an observer (for safety), but she is doing much better.

Her stamina is still low due to the after-effects of the radiation, but she is dealing with it. It does hamper any decision concerning activities away from the house, but we are confident that this will turn around eventually.

Judy has seen the first doctor concerning the ongoing problem with her right leg. He thinks it is a pinched nerve in her back (probably the result of the fall she took while in rehab). He scheduled an appointment with the back specialist and some X-rays to try to pinpoint the source of the problem. We are pleased that this is being addressed.

The lack of appetite is still a problem. The radiologist has assured us that this will pass eventually, but it remains a major concern at this time. Fortunately, she is able to get an instant breakfast down in the morning and an *Ensure* in the afternoon. Other than that, her food intake is limited: cereal (hot & cold), applesauce, toast & jam, ice cream, fruit cocktail, puddings, OJ, milk, and tomato juice. So far, she has been unable to get down any type of meat, fish, or chicken. This has, for the time being at least, eliminated the "Let's go out to dinner" evenings.

When she is not going to one of her many doctor appointments, Judy has expanded her "world" to include the deck where she busies herself caring for her many flowers and plants. The last few days of rain-free weather have necessitated watering those "babies" of hers. This gives her additional practice at walking and hopefully helps to increase her stamina as well.

As always, we thank all of you for keeping us in your thoughts and prayers. We cannot tell you how much that means to us. Thank you.

Earle & Judy

> This is another short note to her friend Lynda. Here, Judy again mentions her stated goal of reclaiming the ability to drive.
>
> This goal gave her a strong reason to push forward. The fortitude this required may have been difficult to muster under any other circumstances.

Wednesday, August 12, 2009

I'm doing OK; the doctors are still baffled with the right leg. I'm going for an MRI on the spine soon. That is the only thing that is keeping me from driving. Still not eating good, but they tell me to be patient, it will come.

I am looking forward to seeing you on the 14th.

Judy

Judy's Journey

As we should have been accustomed by this time, the nature of this update was to take a dramatic change of tenor. Gone would be the casual, relaxed pace. It would be quickly replaced by a sense of urgency and apprehension.

Thursday, August 20, 2009

I know it has been a while, but things were on a fairly even keel until just recently and reporting "no news" simply didn't seem necessary. That has all changed now.

Earlier this week, Judy had a CT scan to determine her current status and map the progress of her recovery. They were assessing her to verify that things were getting back to normal. They did confirm that the Sarcoidosis is gone. It evidently responded to the steroid that has caused so many other problems.

Unfortunately, in addition to that positive news, they did find a spot on her left lung that was not noted in her last scan. This is disturbing, particularly because of the extensive potential possibilities. She saw the pulmonary specialist today. Without any delay, he scheduled her for an immediate bronchoscopy. For our non-medical friends, this is a procedure that sends a fiber optic device into the lung so the doctor can see what the spot truly is, by remote, but direct observation. This is an outpatient procedure, but there is considerable recovery time involved because Judy will need to be anesthetized. For this reason, I will be taking her in for the procedure and expect to have firsthand information to report to you tomorrow.

As always, thank you for all your thoughts, prayers, and continued support.

Earle & Judy

> The follow-up to the anxious message from the previous day is considerably more informational. It still conveys a sense of urgency as the after-effects of the procedure play out. As time goes on, this will become a recurring scenario whenever Judy has some sort of medical procedure. I am placed in the position of the on-scene observer; Judy does fine, but I'm a wreck.
>
> It was her strength and ability to cope with these never-ending situations which somehow enabled me to survive as well. I was drawing strength from her—an accurate description of our entire relationship. She had always been, and continues to be, my personal source of inner strength and fortitude.

Friday, August 21, 2009

What a day! Boy, are we glad this day is now behind us. The procedure went pretty much as planned except that we did not expect it to be such a lengthy ordeal. The actual procedure took about an hour, but there was an hour of paperwork and prep, followed by three hours of recuperation. The camera wasn't able to get to the spot, so they injected some sterile water into the area in question and then withdrew it. The fluid, with any cells in the withdrawn specimen, was then sent to the State Lab for analysis. We should receive the results by Tuesday. The doctor would not speculate as to what it might be, as there are so many possibilities. We had hoped for some more immediate answers, but I guess we will just have to wait.

Following the procedure, we left the hospital just in time to cross the compound and make her 1:30 p.m. appointment at the surgeon's office. This was a follow-up to the recent emergency surgery—we got an A+ on the progress with regard to the healing and our "nursing care" of the wound site following the operation. It was nice to get some answers and immediate feedback.

We are now home, but since our return, Judy's recovery has been a little scary. She has a temp of 102+, a racking cough, even less appetite than before (if that is possible), and she has been asleep since we came home. All of this is within the "normal" parameters that we were told to expect. I have an instruction sheet with several numbers to call and specific criteria to watch for to know when intervention is required. Tomorrow should be better. As it was explained to us, the introduction of the foreign object—the fiber optic tube—causes the body's immune system to react, which is the reason for the fever and other side effects.

As always, thank you one and all for your support. It truly helps to know that there are folks in our corner, especially at a time like this.

Earle & Judy

This next update did not have much to convey in the way of news.   As mentioned previously, I had discovered early on that if I went much more than a week without some kind of report, many of the update recipients would get edgy and become concerned. To avoid undue anxiety, I had learned to limit the gaps between messages to about a week. When longer intervals occurred, some news items, which might otherwise have been perceived as being of minimal significance, were elevated to a reportable level in order to formulate a "satisfying" update (as witnessed here).

Tuesday, September 1, 2009

Not a lot to report, but I don't want you to think we've forgotten you.

Judy had an appointment with the pulmonary specialist this week. All of the results are not in yet, but those that are have been of the good news variety.

They have ruled out a number of things that the problem is not. Some of the "possibilities" eliminated by the bronchoscopy results give us reason to be thankful. We now know that we can exclude such threats as TB and pneumonia. This provides a great sense of relief even though the final report is still in the works.   That will be the definitive analysis of the substances withdrawn with the sterile water (which had been injected into the lung) and then sent for culture. We were told at the beginning that this could take several weeks, so we are not expecting these results for some time.

Judy's stamina is still an issue, but she seems to be getting around the house much better than in recent weeks. I notice little things that she has accomplished during the day while I was at work. I think a nap is still an essential part of the daily schedule, but the overall improvement is evident.

She reported tonight that for the first time in a long time, she was able to actually <u>taste</u> something she was eating for supper. Taste has been absent and has presented a major issue for several weeks now. Hopefully, this trend will continue and lead to an improvement in her nutritional intake.

As always, thank you, each and every one of you, for your continued support, good thoughts, and prayers. Your encouragement has been a source of strength for both of us.

Earle & Judy

Now, a week later, there was much to report. We had been waiting for the results of various tests, scans, and follow-ups. Here, we seize the opportunity to share some of that encouraging news with our supporters. (Could it be possible that I was starting to think of them as our "fans"?) This was a busy time in the continuing treatment of Judy's condition. We were thrilled to be able to convey the combined feelings of relief and hope which we were experiencing.

Tuesday, September 8, 2009

Today was an especially busy day. Judy had two scheduled doctor appointments and an unplanned consultation with her pulmonary specialist. The extra visit was required because the second antibiotic prescribed had the same effect as the first. Not to be too graphic, let's just say that Judy's stomach violently rejected the medication—along with whatever she had eaten recently. As of this writing, we are still awaiting his call to see if he has another plan in mind.

The first appointment this morning was with Dr. K., the radiologist. He had the results of the MRI providing us with confirmation of how effective the "whole brain" radiation treatment had been. We knew that the verdict could have gone either way, so I made arrangements to be there with Judy. The news was the best we could have hoped for.

There is <u>no evidence of any new tumors</u>. This outcome is even more significant because the test was what is referred to as a fine plate scan. If I understood correctly, the scan examined one millimeter slices as opposed to the normal three mm. This provides the doctor with the best possible opportunity for a detailed examination of the affected area. In addition to that good news, the three primary tumors show about a 50% reduction in size. This is a considerable decrease and definitely an encouraging report.

163

Judy's Journey

The determination was made that we now need to follow up with specific spot radiation. This will be a one-time procedure which will focus higher doses of radiation into the core of the three primary tumors. In the best case scenario, the spot radiation would result in reducing them to a minimum size or better still, could potentially destroy them altogether. The doctor has assured us that the procedure is less drastic than the whole-brain treatment and will not require as monumental a recovery. We have started the process and expect to complete this step within the next few weeks.

The second scheduled appointment was with the surgeon, Dr. G. This was a follow-up on the recent gastric surgery and this visit went well. Dr. G. prescribed a new medication to help with Judy's impaired digestive system, but I must add, in general, she was pleased with Judy's progress. We discussed long term possibilities as to the restoration process. *(This is the projected surgery to reconnect the healed sections of the bowel in order to reverse the colostomy.)* She indicated that the longer we were able to wait, the higher the success rate for this procedure. We have reluctantly agreed that it would be wise not to pursue the operation for at least a year to give Judy's system time to regain strength and maximize the chances of a good outcome.

The ongoing complications related to Judy's stamina, appetite, and the right leg deficits are unchanged. We continue to pursue solutions to all of these side issues in an effort to restore some degree of normalcy to Judy's day-to-day life.

As before, thanks to all of you for your continued support. It has been a constant source of strength through all of this.

Earle & Judy

This had been another trying week of treatment and endless adaptation to the new impairments that this deadly adversary had imposed upon Judy. She continued to deal with the ongoing doctors' appointments and treatments as they became part of everyday life and all too common.

Not all of the scheduled activities were due to the treatment of the cancer. Some were normal scheduled events, but they all took their toll on Judy's strength and stamina. Although she never complained, it was obvious that there were times when her resolve was being tested to its limit.

Wednesday, September 16, 2009

Today was a long and busy day. Judy is so utterly exhausted that she is presently sleeping through the Red Sox game—for Judy, that's tired!!

We started the day with an appointment with Dr. J., the neurosurgeon. He explained, in some detail, what the process would be for the next step of treatment: the focused radiation. *(The medical world calls this discussion of risks and benefits "informed consent.")* He confirmed the good results from the whole-brain treatment and outlined the procedure to come. As happened so often during this journey, we were united in our desire to get this next step behind us so we could concentrate on returning to something akin to normal.

Next, we went to the eye doctor. This was the regularly-scheduled biannual visit. Judy's vision has been troublesome lately, but the ophthalmologist has assured her that there is no evidence of cataracts (another possible side effect of the radiation) and that she merely needs a new prescription for her glasses. Now, that is mundane for a change! This has been done, and the new specs should be in next week.

Finally, she had a Herceptin treatment in the afternoon. The doctor indicated that since the Herceptin was apparently doing a good job of protecting her from the spreading of the original cancer, he is planning to continue it indefinitely. This will mean a trip to the oncology center every three weeks, but if it is providing the protection that he seems to feel it is, it will be worth the ongoing appointments.

As we've said so many times, thank you for your ongoing support. We appreciate all the good thoughts and prayers.

Knowing that all of you are in Judy's corner has been a source of strength that we have both been able to draw from.

Earle & Judy

The next two updates, although short, relay some significant news. In the first, we share that the Spot Radiation treatment which has been pending for some time has finally been performed.

The second purports to cover a week's worth of news. It tells of noticeable improvements in multiple areas which have been of concern for considerable time now.

Tuesday, September 22, 2009

Yesterday, the radiation scheduler called and set up the appointment for the final radiation treatment. It was set for 2:00 p.m. today. Judy arranged transportation and went in for the procedure.

The treatment was all that it was built up to be. She was immobilized for almost an hour and a half while the beams of radiation were administered. She was able to get through the session and was home by the time I returned from work.

She is understandably tired. We have a sheet of possible side effects to watch for over the next three days.

Now that the treatment has been completed, the next step will be an MRI in seven weeks. This will be followed by an appointment with Dr. K. a week after that.

Until we get to the follow-up appointment there probably won't be much to report. That is when it will be determined if the treatment accomplished all that it was designed to do.

I can report that Judy is resting comfortably and not displaying any of the adverse side effects on the sheet. She is displeased with the poor showing from the Red Sox, but in good spirits other than that.

Thanks to everyone for your ongoing support. We are more grateful than we can ever tell you.

Earle & Judy

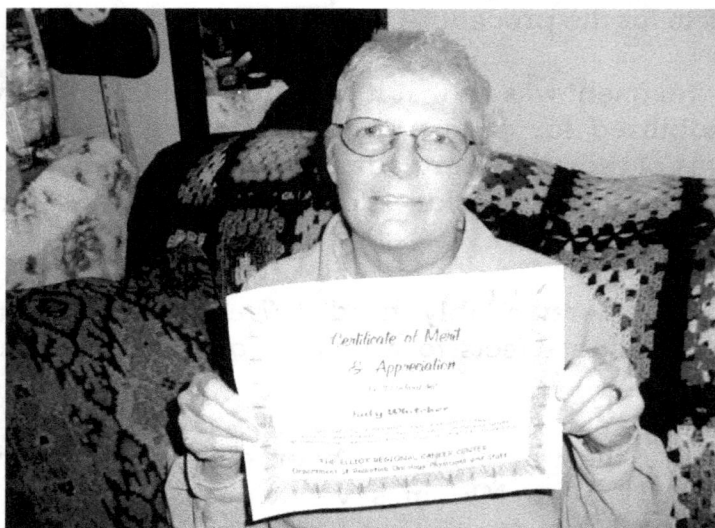

Judy displays her *Certificate of Merit & Appreciation* following her completion of the final radiation treatment.

Monday through Friday, October 5-9, 2009

I'm a little tardy with this update. For some reason, we "turned up the wick" at work this week. (At this time, I was working for a ready mix concrete company. Predictably, the fall brings extended work schedules with the season change.) I have been coming home simply exhausted after putting in some very long days at work.

Judy went to get the results of the leg/nerve tests from last week. She had previously related to me that the tests were much more involved than she had expected. Given a choice, she would not agree to repeat them. In the week between the test and the follow-up, the leg has been showing marked improvement. Judy has regained some of the feeling in it. She is also able to walk much better. The doctor initially listened to Judy's report of these changes, then he broke out his little rubber hammer. When struck, the leg displayed the actual expected, i.e. "normal" reflexes; something that had not been present for several weeks. The doctor was so pleased that he released her to start walking more and to increase activities as tolerated as the improvement continues. He was not able to determine any definite cause for the difficulty, but thought that it could be another side effect of the steroids since they are apparently still wearing off. The bottom line is that conditions are improving.

Judy's appetite and her ability to eat more are also showing marked improvement. While on the surface this may sound like the same thing, it truly reflects progress in two very different areas. She is not only consuming more, but she is now experiencing hunger and has a desire to eat again. This has been absent for some time. We are especially encouraged by this change for the better.

As always, thank you for all your thoughts and prayers. We are sure that we are seeing the results as Judy continues to improve.

Earle & Judy

This short message is one from Judy to her friends and co-workers. It relates her experiences participating in the much-anticipated, local cancer walk. This was a rather large, well-promoted fundraiser in which Judy was invited to take part. She was the focus for her supporting team. This occasion was something Judy had been looking forward to for months. No amount of argument could dissuade her from taking part. Even when the fickle, New Hampshire weather turned especially foul, she was determined to participate in the event.

As we all expected, not only did she join the walkers making the start, she, in fact, completed roughly half of the scheduled course. By that time, the unusual winter-like weather had gotten the best of her and I had to pick her up short of the finish line.

Once again, we were all in awe of her determination and courage. Although she was not able to complete the course, she still viewed it in a positive light and conveyed that thought to her friends in this note. It was another triumph for her.

Sunday, October 18, 2009

I did my cancer walk today in Manchester, NH. The weather was horrible. It rained, sleeted, and snowed. I only made it halfway and Earle had to come and get me because I just couldn't make it. Some of my team was very cold too.

Here's a picture of MY TEAM that walked with me and pushed my wheelchair for me. I'm sitting in my chair wrapped in my blankets trying to get the chill out of my bones, but it was worth it.

Judy

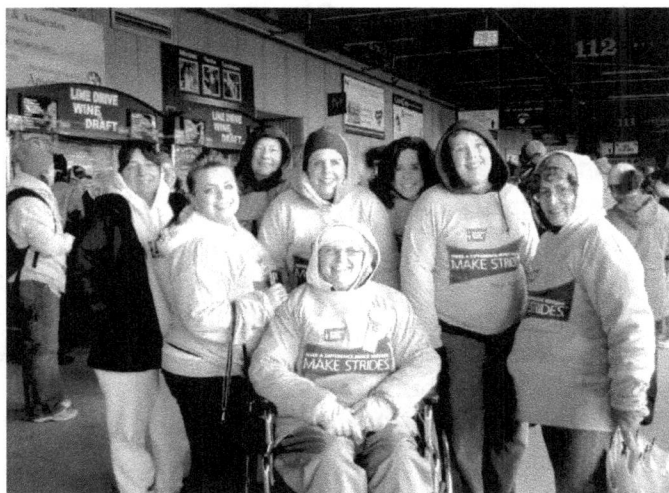

An enthusiastic Judy is surrounded by her TEAM of family and friends:
Jennifer, Cindy, Lynda, Christina, Julie, Andrew, and Rosa
as they prepare to join others for the
"American Cancer Society Making Strides Against Breast Cancer Walk."

Judy's Journey

Now and then, the news is too good to sit on and must be shared as soon as it can be written. Although they do not contain much in the way of news from the medical front, these next two updates demonstrate evidence of such encouraging progress that we felt compelled to get the messages out right away.

During most of the time that Judy was under doctors' care, we would accept any small improvement as a positive sign and a source of renewed hope. What we share here was monumental by comparison. It served to greatly lift our spirits and caused hope for a future—which had seemed so elusive just a few weeks before—to surge once again.

Wednesday, October 21, 2009

This update is going to be a little different. There is no momentous medical news to pass along, but the news is nonetheless significant.

Over the past two weeks, Judy has undergone some remarkable changes in her condition. Her leg, which has been such a source of concern for some time, has suddenly started to recover. As mentioned previously, the doctor thinks the problem may have been related to the side effects of the steroids. The recovery started slowly but has progressed steadily and rapidly. Judy is able to get around much better. Stairs no longer present a barrier. Driving is no longer the problem it once was, in fact, she took herself to an appointment on Monday and ran some errands on Tuesday. I think she has a lunch date for Friday. She is finally able to enjoy her new car. We rejoice in another victory for her!

In addition to the greatly improved mobility, Judy has had a dramatic change in her appetite and eating habits. She now actually has an appetite again! The diversity and quantity of what she is eating has shifted significantly toward what could again be considered normal. There are still some things which do not agree with her recovering taste buds, but the change is encouraging. Her stamina is still somewhat reduced but is showing marked improvement as well. The recent outings admittedly leave her a bit tired—but it's a good tired.

The changes over these past two weeks have been remarkable. We are certain that we are seeing the results of all of your collective prayers and thoughts. We can't thank you enough for keeping us in your hearts. Thank you.

Earle & Judy

Friday, October 30, 2009

This is another non-medical update. The next actual medical information is expected sometime around the end of November. At that time, additional tests will be conducted to assess the effectiveness of the last radiation treatment.

This news flash is intended to catch everyone up on Judy's continuing recovery. She has been experiencing a gradual return to some semblance of normalcy. This past week has been eventful indeed.

On Monday, we went into Judy's workplace to meet with her former co-workers to celebrate her retirement. It was a touching time. We were especially pleased to be joined by our daughter Chris, our son Chuck, and his wife Julie.

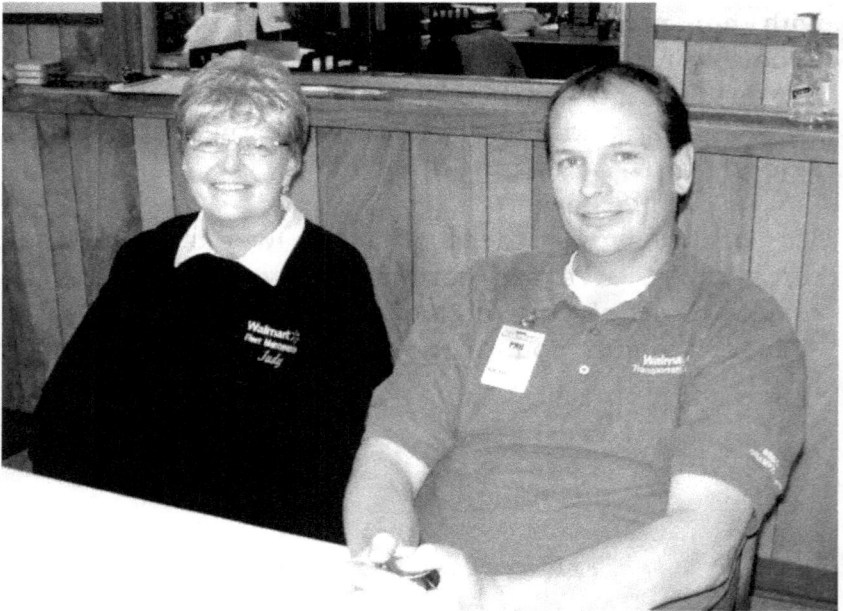

Judy is all smiles at her Retirement Party. She is sitting with Phil, her boss at Wal-Mart.

On Tuesday and Wednesday, we took a short trip to Foxwoods and Mohegan Sun to celebrate my birthday. (These are "Reservation-based" casinos in Connecticut which we enjoyed visiting.) We had a good time.

Although we did not come home with any winnings, we didn't leave everything behind either. Judy thoroughly enjoyed the outing. It was a long-awaited taste of normal life which she desperately needed in order to counteract the endless "patient" existence that she had been living for so long.

On Thursday, Judy had a doctor's appointment and later a dental appointment. She took herself to both. Today, she went into her shop and visited with the other shift of co-workers whom she didn't get to see on Monday.

While she has had an unusually busy week and she is admittedly tired from all the activity, she has been able to withstand the strain of an active week. That is definitely something which she would not have been able to tolerate a couple of weeks ago. We are both encouraged by this progress and can only hope that it continues.

We would like to take this opportunity to once again thank you all for keeping us in your thoughts and prayers. We are certain that you have all played a part in these latest advancements.

Thank you.

Earle & Judy

> Ahh—the roller coaster life of a cancer patient in treatment continues. As encouraging as the past few weeks had been, we are again on that frightening downward spiral which inevitably follows the elation experienced while at the peak of the ride.

175

Judy's Journey

Suddenly, everything that had been so encouraging either stopped or went into reverse. We were back clinging to wisps of hope in a seemingly-endless morass of disappointments and gloomy predictions.

No matter how dark these days became, Judy always stood tall in the face of whatever came her way. Her stalwart determination and strength of character carried her through these difficult times. They were in no small way what enabled me to endure the frustratingly helpless position in which I found myself as well.

Friday, November 20, 2009

For all of you who have been wondering why the updates dried up, the short answer is: to date, there was nothing new to report. That has all changed now, so get your favorite beverage, settle into a comfy chair, and get ready, as this could get wordy.

As of the last communication, I was telling you how much Judy's condition was improving. Then, about a week and a half ago, she hit a plateau. The improvements that we were so pleased to report have stopped altogether and she seemed stuck in place for a while. Then, everything which we had watched improve started to decline. Her newly found appetite disappeared and all she could seem to manage was a single bite of whatever she was having at the time. This continued for a week or so with no visible signs of improvement. We had come to the conclusion that this was another result of the second round of radiation. There seemed to be no alternative, but that we would simply have to tough it out until the effects abated. Throughout this process, she was also losing weight at an alarming rate. The doctors opted not to inundate her system with additional drugs, but rather to monitor the situation and be prepared to step in if required. That time has arrived.

For the past two days, she has been unable to keep anything down with the exception of hot chocolate. We all remain puzzled why this one beverage is so agreeable to her system, particularly since it used to cause her to break out in hives. Last night, I had to get stern (*yeah right*); I insisted that she contact the doctor's office today (Friday). She finally did make the call and they told her to come right in.

They examined her and drew blood at the office. Next, they sent her to the hospital for a test to check for Barrett's Esophagus. This is basically an X-ray of the upper digestive system. They also wanted to rule out any possible blockage. The earlier exam showed that in addition to being severely dehydrated, she has lost almost 20 lbs. in the last few weeks. She has to return tomorrow (Saturday) for a two-hour rehydration treatment. We do not recommend this weight loss program to anyone looking to drop a few pounds. It is just not the way to go.

We are going to be trying some short-term pharmaceuticals (no steroids!); one to speed up her digestive system and another to promote increased appetite. This treatment starts tomorrow. We will let you know if it helps. We certainly hope that it does what it is designed to do and can reverse this alarming development.

As always, we thank each and every one of you for keeping us in your thoughts and prayers. We are certain that you have all had a hand in getting us through what we have conquered so far. We are confident that we will overcome this latest setback and get back on the road to recovery.

Thank you one and all.

Earle and Judy

In the ensuing week and a half since the last update, the conditions have changed again; this time for the better as reported here. One would think that by now, we would have adapted to the manic swings of good news/bad news, but the truth is that we never did.

Each new occurrence brought its own set of elations or disappointments—depending on which end of the pendulum we had swung toward. Every time conditions improved, we hoped that it would be permanent. Each time there was a regression, we prayed that we could overcome it.

Although subtle, these constant changes from high to low can be extremely taxing on the human ability to cope with any given situation. As mentioned earlier, Judy was still exhibiting an unfailingly, positive attitude toward everything. I, on the other hand, was not dealing anywhere nearly as well with the unrelenting flux in which we found ourselves. It was her strength that enabled me to remain a viable contributor to the treatment process. What a strange and foreign world we had found ourselves in.

Tuesday, December 1, 2009

It sure seems to have taken a long time to reach the point where we currently find ourselves. The day has finally arrived for the test that will tell the story of how well Judy's last treatment protocol worked. She went for the MRI yesterday. The follow-up doctor's appointment was today. This consultation could have been either good news or bad news, depending on how effective the radiation was. Judy asked me to be there when we met with the doctor, so I left work at noon today and we went together to see Dr. K., the radiologist.

When he came into the room, he was very upbeat. He wasted no time in telling us that the MRI showed the results for which they had strived. All of the tumors had been successfully reduced in size and showed signs of having been "disrupted." As he explained, the centers of the tumors appeared to be transparent and no longer active.

This is the best outcome for which we could have hoped. At this point, the plan is to follow up with subsequent MRIs; the first, in three months, to monitor the tumors and to be sure that no new, questionable sites appear. After quizzing him at some length, we were apprised as to what to watch for. We are to remain alert for headaches, dizziness, memory loss, and an inability to multitask. It's a good thing that I'm not being monitored—because I never could multitask.

Given the current prognosis, our primary goal now is to concentrate on getting Judy back to a level of health and vigor which will enable her to lead something resembling a normal life again.

We have vacation plans for next year. Now, we have a realistic expectation of seeing them fulfilled.

In addition to this encouraging news, it should be noted that the recently mentioned treatment to overcome Judy's inability to eat has started to show signs of effectiveness. In the last three days, she has gone from eating practically nothing to a nearly normal appetite. She is now eating almost ordinary quantities of food again. The change has been dramatic and genuinely welcome. Her alarming weight loss seems to have stabilized. We will be monitoring her closely to ensure that she starts to regain some of that lost weight so that her body has a cushion with which to combat illness.

We are certain that each and every one of you has had a hand in helping us reach this level of recovery. We know in our hearts that the fact that all of you have kept us in your thoughts and prayers has played a major role in getting us to this point. You have made it possible for us to share with you this, the best of all possible news. Thank you, one and all.

Earle & Judy

While it is true that there is still a full month left in 2009, this was the last update for the year. A combination of events would delay the next update well into the month of January. However, it can be noted here that during this time Judy continued her recovery and healing in the manner of a sine wave on an oscilloscope. There were peaks and troughs, but a relative feeling of cautious relief punctuated this time frame.

The holidays were celebrated in a somewhat subdued fashion compared to prior years, but we celebrated them nonetheless—and with our hearts full of thanks. Judy had always been the dynamo that drove the holiday festivities for us. Now, no matter how brave a front she put on, the simple truth was that she was obviously not up to the level of merriment which had been the hallmark of our revelry in years past. Everyone, even the grandchildren, seemed to understand and accept this. Indeed, we were all just glad that she was able to be with us. This holiday season was marked with a new appreciation of each other.

2010

The New Year's first update starts with an apology and an explanation as to why there has been such an extended gap in the flow of information. Through experience, I had learned that the recipients are a hungry bunch and get restless when they are not provided with a steady stream of reports concerning Judy's progress.

I am certain this is due to their personal involvement, concern, and the love they all feel for Judy. I recognize this and endeavor to keep the updates flowing. This break in the stream of data was primarily due to an all-too-common problem in today's electronic world—a computer bug.

Having finally remedied the problem, this report goes on to relate Judy's continued on-again, off-again progress, but it emphasizes her continued optimistic outlook. This has been her typical attitude throughout her entire life, long before this current health crisis.

Thursday, January 21, 2010

Sorry this has been so long in coming. My laptop was down with a "bug" and I did not want to take a chance of inadvertently sharing it with others. It's returned to service now, with a clean bill of health. We are pleased to be back in contact with the world again.

Judy had an appointment with the cardiologist last Tuesday. This was a regularly scheduled checkup to monitor her tolerance to the continued treatments of Herceptin. As you may recall, one of the long-term side effects is the possibility of impaired heart function. The checkup went well.

All indications are that there has been no change in the test parameters since her last examination six months ago. This is encouraging in that it means that she is tolerating the Herceptin treatments and can continue them. The Herceptin is important because it keeps the cancer in check and prevents its spread to other organs and areas of the body. *(Its chief inadequacy is that, as a large molecule, it cannot effectively cross the blood-brain barrier. This limits its usefulness in preventing brain cancer metastasis.)*

Currently, one of our main concerns is her continually fluctuating appetite. The recent steroid treatment that had been so successful with symptom management has since run its course and is no longer boosting her hunger level. It seems that her appetite has, once again, decreased to a level less than what is desirable. We will be keeping a close eye on this development to be sure that it doesn't get out of hand.

Generally speaking, Judy is maintaining her upbeat approach to everything. I must say that we are having fun with her new hairdo. She calls it the "Jack Nicholson look." I'm not sure Jack would agree, but it certainly is unique. She still experiences a slightly reduced energy level, but we have both learned the benefit of the afternoon nap.

Once again, we would like to take this opportunity to thank you all for your continued support. We thank you for your thoughts and prayers. We also ask that you join us in support and prayer for all who have come under the pall of this insidious disease.

Thank you.

Earle & Judy

Here, less than a week later, we provide another report of busy days filled with doctor visits and checkups. The majority of the news is of a positive nature, all except that continuing problem of Judy's lack of appetite—a condition that will persist throughout this entire ordeal.

Even the everyday non-cancer-related doctor visits were worthy of inclusion in the updates as everyone hungered for any and all reports on Judy's condition. Judy's sense of humor and her innate ability to see the comic relief in any situation is mentioned again as well.

Wednesday, January 27, 2010

Brace yourself—this will be a triple report. It has been a busy week! We have seen the podiatrist and the ophthalmologist and we have also gone in for a Herceptin treatment. For those of you with sufficient capacity to download pictures, I will include a shot of what Judy calls her "Jack Nicholson" look.

The podiatrist took the rest of the nail from the big toe of Judy's left foot. An ingrown toenail, the original problem, had gotten out of control. Her inability to fight off infection has been cause for concern, but everything seems to be back in check now.

The eye doctor had good news. The pressure that they continuously monitor is up slightly, but still well within acceptable limits. Years ago, when this first became an item of concern, it was high on the watch list. These days, it is relegated to back-burner status. It's just nice to know that it's under control and no longer a pressing problem.

Monday, we went for the tri-weekly Herceptin treatment. One part of this process is to consult with the oncologist, Dr. B. He admitted to being a little worried about the current level of Judy's appetite which has continued to decline, but he concluded that keeping a watchful eye on the situation will suffice for now. He was pleased with Judy's overall general progress. He informed us that the Herceptin treatments can continue indefinitely as long as she is able to tolerate them. This means on-going monitoring of a number of items, but at this juncture we are getting used to all of the tests.

The treatment proceeded without any problems. Her stamina level remains impaired, but we have learned that those all-important afternoon naps serve to restore her energy reserves as well as can be expected. Yes, we, is the correct choice of wording since this is one part of the treatment plan that I can monitor in the first person as well. When she naps, sometimes—OK, most of the time—I join her.

As always, we take this opportunity to thank all of you for keeping us in your hearts and prayers. We are sure that Judy's progress and positive response to her treatment is due, in no small part, to all the support we have received.

Thank you one and all.

Now for those who are able to download pictures, I have attached a shot of the new "do." Open at your own discretion.

Earle & Judy

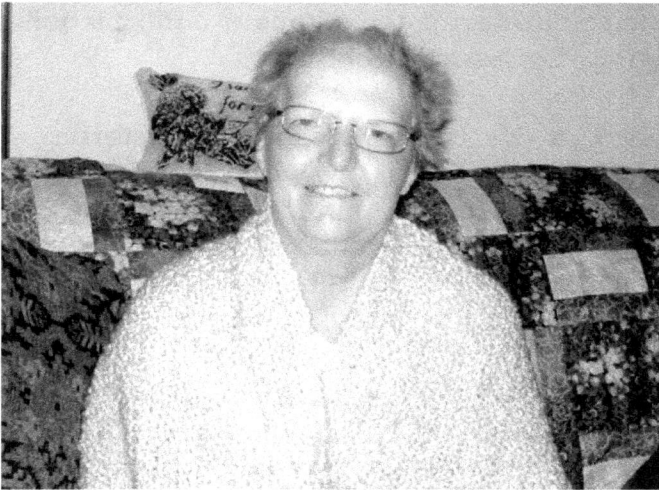

This is Judy's "Jack Nicholson Look."

With almost three weeks about which to report, one would think that there would be an abundant amount of news to relate. At this time, however, this was not the case. Often, we spent the interlude between updates simply living our routine existence, taking care

189

of the daily tasks that define modern life. Through our exposures to the abnormal, we had learned to cherish everything "normal" in our lives. Sometimes, normal is highly underrated.

Tuesday, February 16, 2010

I know that it has been some time since the last update, but frankly, there has been nothing of noteworthiness to report. Since I never intended this to be a report of mundane day-to-day happenings, I have been reluctant to send out updates with no fresh news. In fact, this could be considered the ultimate confirmation of the old saying, "No news is good news."

Judy had a Herceptin treatment yesterday. The observations and reports are worth noting. The biggest news was that she has gained a pound since her last treatment. This truly is good news as it is an indication that her appetite and eating habits have been improving. This has been an ongoing concern for a long time. It is encouraging to know that our unofficial observations that she has seemed to be eating better are corroborated by the evidence verified by the doctor's scale. It would certainly be encouraging to finally put this stumbling block behind us.

Beyond that, everything else seems to be on track. The level of her stamina, although not back to normal, is continuing to improve. This remains our primary concern at this time. Judy is determined to build up her strength sufficiently to be able to enjoy our vacation travel plans for the summer.

In the interim, she is enjoying following the Olympics. She seems to appreciate all of the disciplines whereas I have my favorites. I like the sledding events and I am a big fan of curling. I know, I know, I like the strategy and team control that are unique to the game; I mean, sport.

As always, we want to thank each of you for keeping us in your hearts and prayers. There is no way to measure the help that you all have been. At this time, we ask that you include all of those who are also battling this horrible disease in your prayers as well.

Thank you, one and all.

Earle & Judy

> Although strictly speaking this was not an update on Judy's battle with the cancer, it was still news that needed to be shared. An unusually strong windstorm had passed our way. We wanted to put everyone's mind at ease; we had come through the vigil and were OK. We felt that this was necessary just in case our long-distance friends and family members had seen general reports on the daily news which may have caused them undue concern.

Monday, March 1, 2010

Not the update that you might have been expecting but big news to us. As a result of a powerful windstorm that passed through here last Thursday at about 10:45 p.m., we lost all of our connections via the world of technology. Power was out; the cable and Internet followed suit the next morning. We have been in "survival" mode since Thursday night.

The generator provided the necessities: heat, running water, hot water, fridge and freezer, and some lights. (Thank you, Mr. Honda!) This makes for an adventure on the first day, but it definitely wears thin after a couple of days.

We rejoined the modern world—to the best of our knowledge—about 6:00 a.m. today. We are beside ourselves with a renewed sense of thanksgiving. We also wanted to let everyone know why you haven't heard from us lately.

We are watching the news for the first time in four days and trying to return to normal. That means no more eight-hour "feeding schedule" tying us to the generator. We started calling it "the baby" because it was so demanding. It did the job though, and we are thankful to have had it.

All is well here and we look forward to getting back in touch with all of our friends and family.

Earle & Judy

This message is short, sweet, and to the point. Though there is no major news to share, I have learned throughout this journey that our many recipients get restless if I go too long between updates.

Monday, March 8, 2010

Things are progressing at a much slower pace these days. Although this sounds somewhat negative, it is, in fact, the most positive course of events that we could hope for. It means that Judy's condition has reached a stable point and that she has started her journey on the long road back to something approaching normal— whatever that is. She is still plagued with the reduced appetite and compromised stamina. The doctor has assured us that the levels she is presently at are well within the parameters that would be considered normal at this point in her treatment. Her weight has stabilized and the balance problems do not appear to be increasing in severity.

Her pulmonary doctor met with her last week. The lung problem which he continues to monitor has shown definite signs of improvement. It is one more thing that is no longer an immediate concern. All reports indicate that we need to monitor her progress, but at this time we are optimistically hopeful that we—Judy and I, as well as her healthcare team—are on the right track.

It has been a long, difficult journey and much still needs to be achieved. Only the combination of Judy's strength of will, augmented by all of your prayers, have brought us to this point. Thank you, one and all, for your continued concern, generous display of support, and your prayers.

Earle & Judy

Again, three weeks have elapsed with relatively little to relate, but there is some positive information. We take advantage of this morsel of good news to generate an update.

Passing reference was made to some weather that we have been experiencing. This was done to downplay any concerns that general newscasts might have created in the minds of our supporters. The truth is that we were getting an unusual amount of rain and although the sump pump may have been earning its keep, we were in no danger of any flooding. We wanted to reassure our friends and family as to our relative safety.

Tuesday, March 30, 2010

We have had a couple of busy days irrespective of the "monsoon" that is passing through. Today, Tuesday the 30th, Judy had her follow-up MRI. We will learn the results of that test next week when we see the radiologist. When we were going in for the MRI appointment, we just happened to see her radiologist, Dr. K., in the hallway. He took the time to stop and talk to us right there in the hall. In retrospect, I can't help but wonder if he's like a lawyer and will send a bill for that "consultation." (I don't really think so. He's a great guy.)

Yesterday, the 29th, Judy had her tri-weekly Herceptin treatment. At these sessions, we are also apprised of how things have been going during the intervening period. The primary concern was whether or not she was losing weight due to the ongoing appetite challenges which she, unfortunately, continues to experience. The good news was that she has maintained the same weight she was at three weeks ago. This tells us that even though she is eating at a less than normal level, she is getting enough nourishment to sustain her current body weight. The conclusion which we draw from this confirmation is that it is good news. It is an indication of her body's increasing strength as she fights her way back to something that is, at least approaching, normalcy.

We continue to be cautiously optimistic and increasingly encouraged by every positive milestone we reach. We are pleased to be able to report each success and are resolved to then move on to the next hurdle, whatever it might be. We plan to get through this journey—one step at a time.

We want to thank each and every one of our family and friends for keeping us in their hearts and prayers. We know in our hearts how much that has helped. Thank you, one and all.

HAPPY EASTER!

Earle & Judy

> Here, it has been a mere week following what all would consider to have been an upbeat report. We are compelled to relay the seeds of that which will grow to become another major development in this ongoing saga of strength and courage. At this time, we are faced with what appear to be insurmountable odds.

Judy's Journey

Tuesday, April 6, 2010

Today's visit to the neurologist brought some mixed results. The good news is that the MRI showed no new activity. This indicates that the cancer has not made any new inroads. At this time, it is inactive.

The not-so-good news was that one of the three spots (tumors), which were treated with the focused radiation, shows "something." "Something" means that whatever is happening is unclear at this time. Judy's radiologist has spoken with her neurologist. Together they have determined that the best course of action is to closely monitor Judy's symptoms for any signs of change and follow up with a second MRI in six to eight weeks. They feel that this may explain the ongoing headaches and possibly the balance inconsistencies. The normal treatment at this time would have been to start a regimen of steroids, but given Judy's reaction to steroids in the past, we all agree that it would be best to hold off on that action as long as possible. We won't have any better idea of what is going on until the next MRI is done and has been read.

Thank you all for keeping us in your thoughts and prayers and for continuing this vigil with us through what seems to be a never-ending nightmare. We are committed to seeing this through. Knowing that you are all in our corner is a huge boost to our morale and provides a source of renewed strength.

Earle & Judy

At last, a glimmer of light that brings with it a spark of renewed hope bolstered by a recent scan report. We are greatly encouraged and continue to look forward to that much-anticipated goal of vacation travel plans during the upcoming summer.

Monday, April 19, 2010

Yesterday was Judy's scheduled Herceptin treatment day. It was also the day that we met with the doctor for the follow-up of the recent CT scan. Understandably, this was a meeting that we were looking forward to on many levels. The preliminary evaluations and tests went well. The most encouraging disclosure was that the ongoing weight loss which had plagued her earlier now appears to be under control. We can only take this to mean that her increased appetite—even though only slightly improved—and current intake of food is sufficient to maintain her present body weight. This has been a persistent problem for some time and she is more than happy to be able to cut back on the supplements. I guess *Boost* isn't at the top of her list of favorite foods.

When the doctor came in to complete his assessment, he was full of questions—mostly about the things that you would commonly expect. Once he had satisfied himself that, indeed, things were going well in general; he then informed us that the CT scan had come back with only positive results. It revealed no problem areas whatsoever! In his professional opinion, this confirms that the treatment protocol which we are currently following is the correct one for Judy. He intends to continue with the established plan of action. This means that Herceptin treatments will continue into the foreseeable future, but we are OK with that. We are settled into the routine; we are comfortable with the plan; and we trust the medical judgments of Judy's healthcare providers.

Following such a full day yesterday, Judy was understandably exhausted. We combined the doctor's visit with some other errands and we found ourselves on the go pretty much all day. It was a long day for her, but Judy purposes to increase her daily activity level to enable her to withstand the rigors of the vacation travel planned for this summer. We have had to cancel our vacation plans for the last two years; she is determined not to do so again this year. I think it is good for her to set these personal goals. It not only gives her positive thoughts to occupy her mind, it also gives her something enjoyable and meaningful to work toward accomplishing.

As I have said so many times in the past, we credit all of you with the strength that has enabled us to fight this terrible disease. We are convinced that your continued thoughts and prayers have been an immeasurable help in our ongoing battle. Thank you, each and every one of you, for your generous support and encouragement.

Earle & Judy

In this update the message is clear. The roller coaster ride is not over yet; hang on tight! What follows, over the next few days, can only be described as perplexing, confusing, and frightening. The next chapter unfolds during a visit with friends—and what would prove to be Judy's last excursion behind the wheel of her new car.

Tuesday, April 27, 2010

This won't be a lengthy update, it's just a quick note to notify you all of the latest developments—yes, developments.

Judy has been feeling much stronger lately and has been attempting to increase her activity level in an effort to build up her stamina. Monday, she went to lunch with a couple of her bridesmaids. Yes, they are still in touch after all these years. Everything went well. Tuesday, she was scheduled to have breakfast and do some shopping with a close friend. I suggested that she take a day or two off to recuperate from Monday, but she was determined to go, and so she did. Unfortunately, this did not go well.

Apparently, the breakfast went fine, but at some point while in the store shopping, she began losing her equilibrium and becoming confused. They cut the shopping short and returned to the friend's house where Judy's car had been left. Judy attempted to drive home and was unable to accomplish the trip; in fact, she got lost leaving the driveway. Our friends rescued her and brought her home.

When I arrived home some three hours later, she was so confused, incoherent, and unstable that I immediately called the doctor. The advice was to head to the Emergency Room and have the situation assessed.

Four hours later, she had been examined in the ER and admitted to the hospital for further tests and treatment. It appears that the tumor which had caused the concern at the last MRI (see update of April 6, 2010, regarding "something" that was unclear at that time) has flared up. Medical intervention will now be required to exert control over the "something" that appears to be highly active and out of control at this time.

Judy has started a steroid treatment—with everyone holding their collective breath—understanding that they must closely monitor her for possible adverse effects. The steroids were the source of multiple problems the last time she was on that prescribed treatment regimen (see update of June 24, 2009).

I left her at about 10:00 p.m. after she had been settled for the night. She was still confused and noticeably upset. Hopefully when I see her tomorrow, the steroids will have started to take effect. Once the swelling has been reduced, she may be a little more clear-headed and in better control. I will keep you all informed.

Thank you for all your support.

Earle & Judy

Next, we encounter a somewhat unusual state of affairs. What follows is the first of two updates which went out on the same day. The situation at the hospital was fluid throughout the day. I was removed from the direct information stream during the day while I was at work. It seemed necessary to keep folks informed with what I considered the latest reports when I posted this next message.

The second report followed later. It contained my firsthand observations when I returned from my visit to the hospital after work. The situation was still vague at this point—vague, confusing, and more than a little frightening—because of so many possibilities and so many unknowns.

Wednesday, April 28, 2010 (5:50 p.m.)

I am attempting to do something at which I am admittedly not good—that is multi-tasking. I am in the process of composing an update on Judy's computer (we refer to them as "units") and monitoring the incoming mail on my unit. Oh my!

At this point, all I have to share is secondhand information. I have spoken with Judy's nurse and from what she has told me, it sounds as if there has been some improvement today. The nurse reports that Judy is in and out of cognitive awareness, but is responding much better than she was last night in both understanding and in following physical instructions: primarily, squeezing fingers, raising hands on command, and such.

Also, there are still some problems with eye-hand coordination, but it appears that the treatments are having the desired effect. When I called, Judy was out having the prescribed MRI done. I should have some news about that in the next update.

I will be heading to the hospital shortly. At that time, I will try to glean some additional information and make some firsthand observations of my own. Until then, thank you for all your generous support. I'll keep you informed.

Earle

Wednesday, April 28, 2010 (10:00 p.m.)

I have just returned from the hospital. The news is mixed—nothing real bad, but not as positive as I had hoped. First, to everyone who lives in the immediate area, I must reiterate: no phone calls or visits at this time. While these are not the doctor's orders, my observations confirm that Judy is simply not up to being a participant in any sort of visit at this time.

Though I was there for over an hour and a half, we were able to communicate successfully for only about 10-12 minutes of that entire period. She is so weak that she not only sleeps most of the time—which she obviously needs—but sometimes, even when her eyes are open, she drifts in and out of the conversation. She is so easily distracted that the effort required to hold up her end of the conversation is simply too much for her to handle. She is not 100% sure of her time frame in the hospital either. At one point, she was telling me what happened there yesterday and I reminded her that she was not in the hospital yesterday, not until 8:00 last night. Then she told me that she had an MRI yesterday, but it had only been about two hours prior to our conversation. Please, rest assured that when she is up to having visitors and phone calls I will let everyone know.

The nursing staff reported that Judy had a rough time trying to keep food down today. While I was there, she tried some mac-'n-cheese, but it did not agree with her taste buds. She was able to keep down a cup of vanilla ice cream and some milk. The nurse was pleased with this progress. In retrospect, it amazes me how mundane accomplishments can take on such monumental significance when the body is attempting to recover from some type of assault to the system.

I left Judy some warm socks and a hat just in case she was cold—at times, staying warm has become quite a challenge—but she did not seem to need them, at least not at present. Her roommate must have the same internal thermometer, because between them, they have the temperature set somewhere in the mid-seventies. While I could hardly draw a breath in the room, they seemed to be quite comfortable.

I hope to have more news following the MRI reading tomorrow. Thank you, one and all, for your continuing support. It means a lot to both of us.

Earle

The hospital stay is producing results at such a slow pace; it is difficult to realize that actual progress is being made. Judy's nearly complete lack of awareness is the most disturbing manifestation of the ailment that I have been forced to face to date. It's as though her mind has been taken over (hijacked?) and she is no longer in charge. Little did I realize that, apparently, this was not too far off the mark from what was actually happening.

Thursday, April 29, 2010

For those who are in the know, it is way past juice time. For those who have no idea what that means, please bear with me; it's late and I am tired. (Juice time, for Judy and I, was synonymous with "bedtime.")

Tonight's visit was an improvement over that of yesterday. Judy is still highly confused about some things and is rambling at other times. She can fluctuate between lucid and incoherent in a heartbeat. It is difficult for her to comply with instructions. I directed her to squeeze my finger like the doctor did in the ER and she was able to make a good solid grip—a vast improvement from Tuesday, when she was unable to make the left hand work at all. However, I then had a hard time to get her to STOP squeezing her left hand. No amount of instruction, command, or direct orders could get through to her. I finally held her left hand down, but that resulted in only partial success at best. She did eat some Jell-O and ice cream and also drank some milk. I understand that she had a hard time with her lunch which was grilled cheese and chicken noodle soup. She does not eat bread at all and cannot stand chicken, so this did not come as a great surprise to me. They are working on what she *is* able to tolerate.

The doctor has read the MRI. Unfortunately, since our visits did not coincide, I did not get to talk to him. Judy's awareness is so impaired that she doesn't know if the doctor was in to see her or not. She still has a long way to go, but today's improvement was encouraging, particularly after last night's disappointing—and I would add, heart-wrenching—visit. We (yes, we did talk about this) both agree that it would be best to hold off on calls and visits for at least one more day. If she continues to improve tomorrow at the pace she moved forward today, perhaps she will be up to a few calls and some quick visits over the weekend.

I must ask that anyone who, even remotely, thinks they may be coming down with any kind of bug, please hold off on in-person visits until you are completely recovered.

Thanks to all of you for your gracious concern and unwavering support. We are grateful beyond description. Together, with your help and Judy's strong will to fight, we will get through this.

Earle

Suddenly, as if a veil had been lifted, clarity and purpose return to our patient. I guess the medical answer is that the low-dose steroids finally took effect. Whatever the reason, I went to the hospital for this visit with a heavy heart and lowered expectations. After the visit, I was so encouraged that when I came home, I was able to compose this update which has a decidedly upbeat lilt to it.

Judy's Journey

The manic course, which this ailment has taken during the last two or three days, has been nothing short of astounding. By this time, we should have been accustomed to these wild changes. In truth—we never fully adjusted to them.

Judy's ability to bounce back from what seemed to be the brink of despair to nearly normal again was simultaneously amazing, confusing, and encouraging. Remember that roller coaster ride I mentioned—the description is certainly apropos.

Friday, April 30, 2010

First things first! Thank you everyone for your prayers for Judy's well-being. And now, the best news of all— ***JUDY IS BACK!!***

Our combined prayers have been answered. Tonight's visit was so different from last night's that I am at a loss for words to adequately describe it. It is such a cliché, but it is so true: "What a difference a day makes."

Tonight when I arrived, Judy was awake, alert, fully cognizant of her surroundings, and 100% in control. She was able to eat some of her meal and was in good spirits. We talked about everything, including what goals we need to work toward so she can be discharged and return home. This conversation could not possibly have taken place on Thursday night. In addition to all of the more serious talk, we were joking and laughing like we usually do. When I heard her laugh, I knew we were back on track.

While I was there, the doctor who sees her when she is in the hospital came in. He is called a "hospitalist." Try to say that quickly three times in succession. He is the oncologist's eyes and ears while Judy is in the hospital. The oncologist does not come to the hospital. He depends on the hospitalist's observations and input to form conclusions about his patients while they are hospitalized. Based on the hospitalist's documentation, Judy's oncologist can then formulate a discharge plan which would be initiated following her release from the hospital. I secretly think of him as Dr. B.'s avatar.

When he entered the room, he could not contain his excitement as he noted the miraculous change in Judy's condition. He informed us that the present plan is to continue with the current treatment, at least through the weekend.

There is a major meeting scheduled for Tuesday. Judy will be the central character and the main topic of discussion. The focus of that consultation will be for them to all put their heads together to devise the final plan for her treatment. The hospitalist said that Judy's job in the interim is to get stronger, try to improve her diet, and be ready to go home when the time comes. She was wholeheartedly enthusiastic about the "go home" part.

To everyone in the area: we feel that Judy is now able to have visitors for short periods, but only in small groups. At this time, we would ask that you do not call on the phone as she is still a little awkward when trying to answer it.

Judy's Journey

We must emphatically remind everyone, please do not stop in if you suspect that you may be coming down with something. Judy is still in a weakened state of immunity and susceptible to any "bug" that might find its way into her compromised system. She is at the local hospital in the city, in Room # (omitted).

As I said in my initial greeting, thank you, one and all, for your prayers and support. We know in our hearts that you have all had a part in Judy's amazing turnaround. We cannot thank you enough.

Earle

From all observations, it would seem that once the recovery started, the pace kept accelerating, not unlike a runaway snowball headed downhill. The medical folks undoubtedly attributed this to the medication and their skill. We were certain that in addition to their abilities, there were other forces at work. Regardless of how, or why, the progress was amazing and once again, we were greatly encouraged.

Saturday, May 1, 2010

Another day and we have more remarkable recovery news to report. The doctors think they are wholly responsible, but we know they are only part of the reason. Judy is keeping her food down—what little she is able to eat. Unfortunately, the loss of appetite and lack of hunger have returned. These appear to be part of the steroid side effects. She is trying to get as much nutritional intake possible as she knows those *"Ensures"* are lurking just around the corner if she doesn't maintain an acceptable level of nourishment.

Our daughter, Chris, stopped by while I was there today and it quickly became apparent that Judy was sufficiently recovered to gang up with Chris at my expense. After what we have just been through, I was more than happy to be the object of their jokes.

She is now able to get out of bed "with an assistant." She asked me to help her to the bathroom today, but by the time I got up and started around the end of the bed to "assist," she had already gotten out of bed and was closing the bathroom door. I am not sure how I was of any help; I couldn't keep up with her. My guess is that she will be home soon and will probably have to do some sort of outpatient rehab to regain some of her strength and motor skills. She may also need some help with coordination and balance as well. We haven't talked to the doctor about this yet, but it would seem to be a logical next step.

Tuesday is set to be a pivotal day in this latest adventure. That is when all of her doctors will sit down together and work out a manageable treatment plan for this newest development. We are not sure in what direction they will decide to go, but Judy, in her usual "positive mode," is already making arrangements to move forward with all of our vacation plans for this summer.

She is somewhat goal-oriented. OK, so "somewhat" may be a bit of an understatement.

I would be remiss if I did not thank you all again for your continued support and prayers. I need to thank you all for putting up with my ramblings as well. These updates have had a dual benefit. Not only have they served as a way for us to keep our family and friends informed of Judy's progress, they have also provided an emotional outlet for me. They have permitted me to unburden myself of the strain and the feelings of helplessness which have so often intruded while we have been traveling this bumpy and convoluted road.

Thank you one and all.

Earle

As the weekend comes to a close, I outline not only Judy's continued progress, but some interesting ways of solving her dietary dilemmas. Evidenced here is the method that became pretty much the standard manner of solving those quirky food issues which became more prevalent than we could ever have anticipated. We simply let her have her own way. Judy ate whatever she liked and found she could tolerate. The subject of returning home was starting to become a topic of discussion at this point as well.

Sunday, May 2, 2010

The weekend has passed and Judy continues to make incredible improvements. She has found the items on the hospital menu which she likes and is able to eat. I watched tonight as she devoured her fish and mashed potatoes. The biggest problem she has is with the lunch menu. It is made up mostly of sandwiches and salads. Judy doesn't do well with bread and is restricted from eating fresh vegetables. She has solved the conundrum by simply choosing ice cream and milk for lunch.

Her motor skills and coordination are improving. She is still falling a little short of what we would call "normal" for Judy, but she is rapidly approaching a point of recovery which we are hopeful will be sufficient to convince the doctor that she is ready to go home. As yet, we have not asked that question, but expect to raise the subject next week.

Judy had several visitors today while I was there. She seemed to handle the extra strain of socializing well. She remained awake, alert, and connected with everyone there. The other thing she has determinedly mastered is answering the telephone. She can now take phone calls if anyone wishes to call. The best way to reach her is to call the hospital at (omitted). When the operator answers, ask for Room # (omitted), Bed 1. That will ring directly to the phone at her bedside.

As always, thank you for your continued support and prayers. We have now seen what can happen with the concentrated effort of many who are determined to make a difference. Thank you one and all.

Earle

Even a one day lapse in the update flow has been known to cause a great deal of consternation among the recipients, particularly during times of crisis. A little reassurance is needed to alleviate their concern.

A major new development is awaiting them in this brief, but important message.

Tuesday, May 4, 2010

For those who were wondering what happened to yesterday's update, I'll just quickly say that this is again proof positive of the old adage: "No news is good news." Judy continues to improve at a slow but steady pace. Until now, there have been no major changes to report. Today however, is a completely different story.

The Tumor Board participants had their consultation meeting this morning. They agreed, by a margin of two to one, to go ahead with brain surgery. The tests indicate that removal of one of the tumors would remediate, or at least improve, Judy's condition. The board members believe that debris from the largest tumor is becoming active and is the culprit causing the latest problems that Judy has been experiencing. We are both in agreement and in favor of the surgery option. As of today, we do not have any specifics: such as a prospective date, what to expect for an outcome, or a recovery time frame. We are hoping that Dr. J., the neurosurgeon, will be in contact with Judy tomorrow to either set up a consultation or to inform her of the proposed schedule. As soon as we have additional information, we will let you all know what the plan is. Though we are, understandably, apprehensive about the upcoming surgery, we are both pleased that we now have a plan to follow. As we understand it, this is far from a routine procedure. The one reassuring element is that we have had dealings with Dr. J. in the past. (Dr. J. performed the original brain tumor excision of the non-cancerous lesion which had affected Judy's vision in 2003. This account has been retold in greater detail in the *Prologue* of *Judy's Journey*.) He is among the medical and surgical experts who comprise that elite group which can truly be called "the best of the best." Though we do not count ourselves fortunate to be facing neurosurgery (again), we consider ourselves unquestionably fortunate to be under his care.

We also recognize ourselves to be equally blessed for being the recipients of all of your prayers and encouragement. You have all contributed so much to Judy's ongoing battle in this seemingly-endless struggle. I cannot tell you how much your support has meant to both of us. Thank you once again.

Earle & Judy

> Just one day later, not only is there news, but there is also a schedule for the recently discussed operation. We are both surprised and pleased—and yes, we are experiencing what would be normal apprehension given the situation—that this next major hurdle will be dealt with expediently. In retrospect, this should have been a signal to us as to the seriousness of the situation, but we were just happy to be free of those irritating delays which so often interrupted the medical process.

The rapidly approaching summer plans are mentioned here as well. They are less than two months in the future now and we are both anxious to see them come to fruition. Now, weighing in the balance are our arrangements to attend a reunion with friends from the military. This is a regularly-scheduled event in which we have been participating for more than thirty years. The travel plans are a driving force in Judy's goal-oriented recovery process. She desperately wants to see these folks one more time.

Wednesday, May 5, 2010

I have just returned home from the hospital. Things are quickly moving forward toward Friday afternoon when Judy's surgery is scheduled. Dr. J. explained the procedure to Judy this morning, informing her of what to expect. According to him, the recovery process should only involve a few days in the hospital following the surgery. She will, of course, need additional recovery time at home. He does not see any reason for us to change our plans to attend the upcoming reunion in Alabama. That is good news indeed as Judy has been counting on this trip for a long time.

Recently, Judy reported a series of strange episodes of visual illusions—very bizarre, indeed. She is apparently experiencing visual anomalies which, by her description, appear to be hallucinations. She describes them as hologram-like visualizations. She also reports sighting *Muppet*-like characters that peek in at her doorway; fish swimming by; and strange puffs of drifting steam or smoke. Dr. J. informed us that hallucinations are another of the potential side effects of the steroids. It is also one of the reasons he wants to move ahead so quickly with the surgery. We are relieved to finally have a plan in place and a specific course of action that will, hopefully, quickly close this particularly disturbing chapter of Judy's ongoing problems.

We thank all of you for your continued support and prayers. We are convinced that you have all had a hand in getting us to this point. Now we need to put this new hurdle behind us. I know you will all be with us in your thoughts and prayers during these next few days. I will let you all know the outcome as soon as I can. Thank you once again.

Earle

Due primarily to the seriousness of the pending operation, but also to keep our concerned readers informed and to help relieve some personal stress and tension, I sent out this otherwise extraneous message. Sometimes, just sharing is helpful. (I have, since, been informed that written expression can be therapeutic.)

Remark: Take special note of the date of this update. The very first communication was dispatched to our friends and family on 5/6/08; the first radiation treatment was scheduled for 5/6/09; today, Judy is recovering from an emotionally-destabilizing event and preparing for brain surgery on the following day. Throughout *Judy's Journey* certain dates seem to have made a habit of recurring prominently with significant incidents.

Thursday, May 6, 2010

Everything is on track for tomorrow. Judy is upbeat and ready for the big day. As I understand it, she will have a special MRI to provide the surgeon with a current, extremely-detailed view of the affected area. This will enable him to target the offending tumor with accuracy and precision. As a layman, this seems logical, even to me. I don't think they want to get in there and make any unexpected discoveries. A current "map" seems to make perfect sense. If all goes as planned, she will be going to pre-op about noon and into the OR an hour or so later. The neurosurgical procedure is expected to take about an hour and a half. I have made arrangements to get out of work early. It is my intention to be there when the doctor meets with Judy just prior to the main event.

We are both highly optimistic and confident that this is going to make a big improvement in Judy's overall well-being. We have the highest regard and faith in the surgeon and we know that all of you are in our corner as well. Thank you for all your support. The next update should include the results of the operation.

Earle

I had promised an update following the surgery. Unfortunately, the full update would have to wait an extra day due to the lateness of the hour. Still, I knew I had to send something or risk causing undue concern among our friends and family.

Friday, May 7, 2010 (actually sent May 8, at 1:30 a.m.)

It is much too late to go into details. Tomorrow, I will make up for the brevity—for sure—but I want to let you all know that everything went great today. Judy came through the operation like the trooper that she is. By the time I left, she had regained consciousness and was already starting to make plans and to give me instructions. The doctor reported that all went as planned without any unexpected hitches. Rest assured that all is well. More details tomorrow—I promise.

Earle

Saturday, May 8, 2010

OK, it has been only one full day since the surgery and things are looking up again. Judy has graduated from the ICU and is now in a recovery room on the 7th floor: Room (omitted), Bed #1. Quite understandably, she is still "a little weak in the knees." She reports that the incision on the back of her head hurts enough that she has difficulty finding a comfortable position to sleep. The nurses are able to provide her with pain meds when she needs them. She is back to a regular diet and her appetite is now quite substantial. When I was apprised of what she had eaten for the day, I was amazed at the quantity of food that she is now consuming. I hope Judy's appetite stays this robust when they get her off the Decadron (the steroid they have been administering to her). Judy is mobile again. She is walking with the aid of a walker, but I think that is just a standard hospital precaution. We went for a walk: once around the floor, and she seemed to do fine. She admits to feeling a bit unsteady. As strong as she was a day before the surgery, I have to think this is just a temporary decline brought on by the anesthesia.

She is still a little foggy about some things, but has all the right answers for the nurses when they stop in. We have not asked the one question on everyone's mind; when will they release her to go home? Since we haven't asked, we have no firm answer, but we tend to think that Tuesday is not an unrealistic target date based on the pre-op discussions we had with Judy's neurosurgeon. We should know more after the doctor checks her progress on Monday.

I can't say this enough: "Thank You" for your continued support and prayers. Look what we have done again, together.

Gratefully yours,

Earle

The good news continues. I confirmed for all the wonderful report of Judy's rapid progress following the operation. The change is so astonishing that I felt compelled to comment on it in detail. It's always a pleasure to convey good news and this is so uplifting that I was eager to share it with everyone.

E. *Whitcher*

Sunday, May 9, 2010 ~ Mother's Day

One piece of news which I have to report is that Judy
has changed rooms again. She is now in Room #
(omitted). It's a private room so she no longer has a
roommate. She has had all external connections (IV's,
etc.) removed. She is still walking around the floor with
someone to watch and assist as needed. They are in the
process of tapering and eventually stopping the
steroids. Good news there! The surgeon informed her
this morning that if she passes the requirements of the
oncologist, as far as he is concerned, he could release
her to go home as early as Monday.

There may be some PT required to regain the strength
in her legs, but it "looks so good following the removal
of the 'mass,'" as he calls it, that he is comfortable with
her discharge. This will still have to get the final
approval of her principal doctor: the oncologist. I guess
there is a strong chain of command in the medical field.

The incision is still causing her some discomfort, but
she is learning to deal with it and the pain meds are
available, as needed. The staples are scheduled to be
removed next week. That, in itself, should make things
less bothersome.

I have no doubt that all who read these updates have
been following Judy's progress closely. Nevertheless, I
feel the need to emphasize that those of us who have
witnessed Judy's transformation are nothing short of
amazed! She went from a totally disconnected,
confused, and incoherent patient, dependent upon
others for virtually everything, to the nearly self-

sufficient, confident individual who now freely and accurately discusses her treatment with complete understanding.

Perhaps those of us who know of all of your contributions understand the transformation a little better. This has been a firsthand display of what is possible with the combined efforts of the medical profession and the power of all of your unselfish and most generous prayers.

As always, I wish to pass along our sincere thanks to all of you for your support and prayers. Know in your heart that your efforts have given us the hope and strength to continue the fight. Thank you one and all.

Earle

Today, I was able to share the news that we had all been waiting for—Judy's return home. While this is always a welcome event, there were some reservations and concerns. None of them, however, could diminish the excitement which we were feeling at having weathered this latest crisis and emerging triumphant at its conclusion. To say that we were euphoric would be an understatement.

The reference to the altered subject line entry calls attention to the fact that normally, I put the numerical designation for the date, such as 5/10/2010, in the subject line of the updates I sent out. Today, the change was such a dramatic improvement that I needed some way to punctuate the positive turn of events. I wanted to capture recipients' attention immediately, so I decided to write the date longhand and place it in the subject line for added emphasis.

Monday, May 10, 2010
Subject: Five, Ten, Two Thousand Ten

Did you notice something different in the subject line? Well that's not all that's different. I'll give you three guesses—and the first two don't count—to see if you can figure out who is at home sitting in her favorite chair.

Yes, the doctors all agreed to send her home a little early with surprisingly few restrictions to complete the healing process. She has to meet with the surgeon in 10-14 days to have the staples removed and to allow him to assess her progress. The next few days are going to be a little hectic as she gets caught up with her other appointments, but the bottom line is— <u>Judy Is Home</u>.

Her walking is still a little hesitant and the doctor emphasized that she is NOT to drive. Other than a lifting limit and no carrying things up or down stairs, she is fairly free to go about her business—of course, with the "as tolerated" caveat.

I can see a hint of a problem in getting her to ease into her old schedule rather than jump in with both feet as she is so apt to do, but I expect she'll soon learn her limitations and abide by them.

This should conclude the daily reports. I plan to continue keeping you all updated, but not on a daily basis, unless of course, there is something newsworthy to report. As always, thank you for your continued prayers and support. I really cannot express in words how much it has meant to us both.

Earle & Judy

A full week has passed. In the following update, we share the medical information received at Judy's post-surgical follow-up. The P.A. provided us with the surgical outcome while removing the staples.

Here, we also learn the outcome of the pathology findings regarding the tumor that was excised. While the staple removal went well, the rest of the story was certainly a cause for concern.

The pathology report detailing the nature of the tumor is quite distressing. The roller coaster ride continues as we hang on tenaciously.

Monday, May 17, 2010

Today, the staples were removed from Judy's incision. I heard a couple of "ouches" during the process, but generally, it went well. The wound is healing nicely and looking much better than it did a week ago. The P.A. checked the standard things: strength, reflexes, and walking. Based on all indications, Judy is recovering from the surgery as expected. Her overall progress is encouraging.

We had expected to be meeting with the neurosurgeon. As it turned out we saw the P.A., because the "boss" was on vacation. We had several questions lined up. Though the P.A. had to leave the room for a while, when she returned she answered our queries. The biggest news she had for us was that the tumor which was removed was, in fact, cancerous. Based on the pathology report, the recommendation was that we contact both our radiologist and oncologist in order to get their opinions about what course of action was best to follow. We have messages out to both doctors' offices and are waiting for callbacks as to what they advise. The P.A. did emphasize that the surgeon was certain that he had successfully removed ALL of the offending mass. Until we hear otherwise, we are focusing on the positive points we learned today.

We will keep you all up-to-date as this latest development plays out. As always, thank you for your support, prayers, and good wishes. We are still in this fight and expect to see it through.

Earle & Judy

More than a week has passed and we finally have something to report. That is not to say that nothing has been happening in the interim, just that we didn't have news for "our readers" as we have begun to think of them.

If the daily stress of not knowing what was happening to her was weighing on Judy, it was not openly apparent. Here, we learn of the new medicine she will be taking. Our knowledge of it and its purpose is somewhat unclear, but we are determined to follow through with whatever course of action extends any realistic degree of hope and promise to us.

Tuesday, May 25, 2010

We met with the radiologist today. Even though his assignment basically ended when the radiation was complete, he still has a stake in Judy's treatment. He also remains "in the loop" as an expert and consultant when her situation is discussed whenever the tumor board convenes for their "roundtable" caucuses. He confirmed what we pretty much knew about the cancerous tumor which had been removed. True to form, he tested and checked all of the usual things that seem to be ubiquitous when a doctor comes into the exam room.

What struck us both though was his inability to disguise his elation with Judy's recovery from surgery and her major overall improvement since the recent tumor removal. We took this to be an encouraging sign. He also assured us that while they would not use additional radiation as a first response, should the situation arise and it would be deemed appropriate, it was still one of the backup plans in reserve. It is good to know that we have not exhausted all of the possible weapons in this battle.

Judy started a new medication today, something called Tykerb (it's Google-able). We were given some insight on how it is expected to work—what is otherwise known as "mechanism of action." If we understand correctly, it is going to replace the tri-weekly Herceptin treatments. We will confirm whether or not that is the case when we see the oncologist on June 2nd. The radiologist also explained that the new drug is a small molecule which they believe will help protect the brain from further invasions by the roaming cancer cells. It just remains to be seen how well she tolerates the new med. Apparently, it is some pretty strong stuff. We are hopeful that she will be able to deal with it well enough to continue with our travel plans for the summer.

It may seem redundant to keep saying this, but we truly mean it when we say thank you for keeping us in your hearts and prayers. There is no doubt in our minds that you all have had a hand in Judy's ability to bounce back from a seemingly-endless deluge of setbacks and "surprises." We are sincerely grateful for your continued support.

Earle & Judy

Now, we are just past the Memorial Day holiday weekend and what we had termed "our test trip." That was a long weekend excursion to New Jersey to visit friends and also to determine if we were able to deal with the logistics and requirements of Judy's new situation. Between the cancer treatment and all of its possible effects, and the many colostomy care considerations, we faced a number of challenges. We were apprehensive about the outcome of this trip because our more extensive plans for the reunion, as well as the long-anticipated summer travel to visit family in North Carolina, would hinge on the results of this three-day outing.

In this update, we also report on our latest visit to the oncologist. Additionally, we share our increased awareness and understanding concerning the new treatment Judy was undergoing. Little did we anticipate the far-reaching ramifications this treatment would have in the near future.

Wednesday, June 2, 2010

Lots to report, so I'll get right to it. First of all, we did complete our scheduled trip to N.J. over Memorial Day weekend. (Thanks again to Madeleine & Jeff for their gracious hospitality.) This trip showed us that we—meaning Judy—can, in fact, make a trip and deal with all of the challenges of the current circumstances. (The colostomy has definitely added a new array of intricacies to all outings—be they brief or extended.) The present situation precludes Judy from driving and restricts her to the position of navigator. Tongue in cheek, I must admit that it is a job for which she is well-qualified as she is quite adept at telling me where to go. We made it down and back in good order and had a great time while there. As it turns out, I may have been a little overly apprehensive, but since this was our first time away from home and the security of established routines, I was not sure what to expect. As I should have known, Judy was the stalwart traveler; just as she has been the outstanding patient these past two years. The encouraging positive results from this trip have convinced us that we will be able to take part in our planned reunion later this month.

Today, we saw the oncologist. He is the one who changed the treatment plan and started Judy on Tykerb.

We had many questions for him and he did his best to answer them all. For the present time, he has prescribed this treatment protocol in place of the ongoing Herceptin which she had been receiving. Once he finds out how well she is able to tolerate the Tykerb, he hopes to add something called Xeloda. This is another powerful drug, similar to Tykerb, with the same disruptive mechanism of action aimed at eradicating rogue cells. If she is not able to handle the combination (of Tykerb and Xeloda), he plans to reintroduce the Herceptin along with the Tykerb. Needless to say, it is quite a juggling act that he is involved with here. He states that each patient is different and has unique reactions to these new drugs. Some trial and error is required to determine which protocol or combination works best.

We are encouraged by this new effort to attack and subdue the brain cancer. The doctor reminded us of the seriousness of the situation—he as much as urged us—to take full advantage of this "good time" to undertake those things which we want to accomplish in our lives—while we still can. It is good advice that we have heard before, but may not have fully taken to heart in the past. I can assure you that we are doing so now.

Judy's Journey

As always, we offer our sincere thanks to all of you for keeping us in your hearts and prayers. We are grateful for your support and cannot say "Thank You" enough.

Earle & Judy

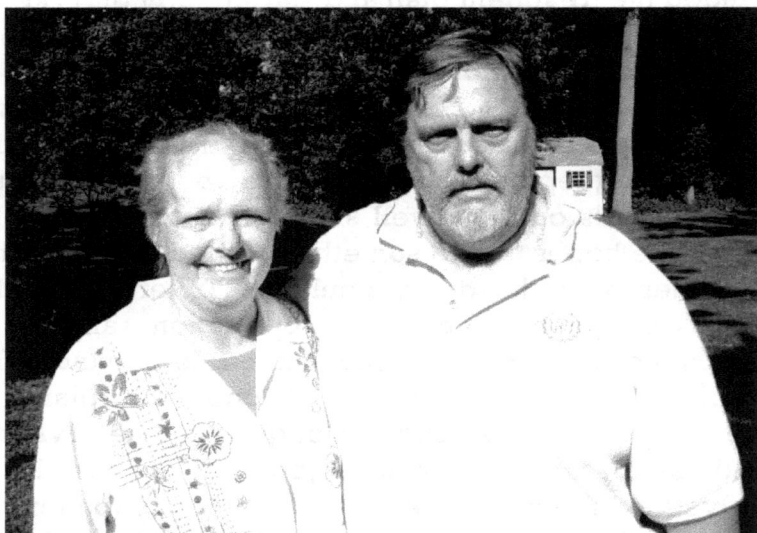

Memorial Day 2010
Judy and Earle successfully negotiated the challenges of their "Test Trip."

In the intervening three weeks-plus between these updates, we have spent most of our time adapting to the new medical protocol that the doctor had initiated.

There is little mention of it in the messages, but the new medication caused substantial disruption to Judy's digestive system. Though challenging, we are adapting to the situation. Initially, it caused her a great deal of discomfort and embarrassment. With the invaluable help of *Imodium*—in our case, truly a miracle pill—we were able to deal with the difficulties the Tykerb caused and managed to lead something akin to an ordinary lifestyle.

We are preparing for the upcoming reunion. This will involve several days of travel to and from Alabama. We are positive and upbeat about doing whatever it takes to make this happen. This event has been a central focus in our lives for more than thirty years. The idea of missing it is simply out of the question.

Saturday, June 26, 2010

I realize it's been a while since the last update, but the fact is there hasn't been anything newsworthy to report. Since our last installment, Judy has met with her oncologist, the pulmonary specialist, and the neurosurgeon, in that order.

We have learned that the oncologist is pleased with her progress and has started the new treatment with an oral form of the chemotherapy agent called Tykerb. If she tolerates that well, he will add the second med that has shown the best results when combined with the Tykerb. They are both quite potent and require some getting used to. So far, she has done well on the Tykerb. I expect the doctor will be trying the combination soon. The lung doctor has been watching a potential problem with one lung. We think this is a result of the original radiation treatment. The spot he has been monitoring hasn't changed and Judy shows no signs of pulmonary distress, so he gave us a thumbs-up at this time.

The follow-up with the neurosurgeon was interesting. He was the doctor who removed the brain tumor which was most recently causing such a fuss. He was so pleased with the recovery that he said he will not need to see us on a recurring basis. He will keep in touch with the other doctors and monitor Judy's progress through them.

All of the medical specialists have given us a green light for our upcoming vacation travel plans. We will be leaving this Wednesday, June 30th. We are looking forward to seeing everyone at the reunion we will be attending.

As an interesting aside, our oldest granddaughter is currently in the hospital. We expect that she will make us great-grandparents either tonight or tomorrow. "And the beat goes on ~."

As always, thank you, one and all, for the precious gift of your prayers and for your continued support. We are truly grateful.

Earle & Judy

What follows is a brief description of our trip to Alabama to attend the reunion of military friends. The narrative is succinct and was solely intended to put the growing number of readers of our experiences at ease and to assure them that Judy was traveling well. The reference to "Hahnites" is simply how we came to refer to ourselves due to the fact that we had all been stationed at Hahn Air Base while serving overseas in Germany. That connection, from forty years prior, has been the basis for these lifelong friendships and is the primary reason that this reunion was so important to both of us.

There were no updates sent out from the reunion itself as we were busy getting reacquainted with our friends from the military. Everyone had a tendency to fawn over Judy, so much so that we ended our days worn out, but in a good way.

The reunion trip was an unqualified success. It helped to lift both of our spirits, particularly after such trying times leading up to this point. Though reality was just around the corner, we savored these few days free of its unrelenting grip.

Tuesday, June 29, 2010

Well, when my employer gave me an unexpected day off today (due to a reduced workload) I think they thought they might hurt my feelings. The truth is they could not have given me a better gift. It gave us an unanticipated early start for our travels. We have put about 470 miles of our trip behind us and are presently ready to get between the sheets in Chambersburg, PA (south of Harrisburg). After looking over the maps, I think we can do the same thing tomorrow and wind up in the vicinity of Knoxville, TN. That will leave us only about 200 miles to cover at our leisure in order to arrive at our destination at the appointed time. Sometimes things just work out.

Happy Trails!

Earle & Judy

Wednesday, June 30, 2010

Greetings from East Knoxville, Tennessee! We accomplished our planned mileage for the day. It put us right where we expected.

We are settled in for a good night's rest with 942 miles behind us and less than 200 miles to go tomorrow. Don't you just love it when a plan comes together?

We have spoken to some of the other reunion-bound "Hahnites" and it looks like everyone else is on track as well. This should be a banner event. I just have to convince Judy that it's OK for her to nap in the car. She feels like she has to stay awake to be company for me. I told her that I'll wake her up if I need her navigational skills. She should get a good night's rest tonight. We are under no pressure to get up and hit the road early tomorrow.

From the road ~

Earle & Judy

This installment went out following our return from Alabama. It starts off with the, now typical, medical and general condition report. The latter part of the message is a thumbnail sketch and an accounting of the reunion itself.

I am still amazed that so many of our friends and family want to hear these mundane reports of our daily existence. Over time, I have come to realize that these updates are their connection to Judy and her valiant battle against the cancer that is constantly trying to deny her a normal life. They have shared our joy in each victory. They have also upheld us during each challenge.

Monday, July 12, 2010

Today, Judy saw the oncologist and our family doctor as well. The oncologist determined that she was tolerating the Tykerb well enough to start the companion pill, Xeloda. I expect this will be initiated in the next week or so. We are gearing up for the next round of side effects and the challenge of finding a way to deal with them. The oncologist also started her on an antibiotic in anticipation of her upcoming dentist appointment.

Apparently, the possibility of an infection must always be considered even when a simple dental procedure is to take place. Everything else, except for a slight loss of weight, checked out OK. He gave her a liquid medication that is intended to help increase her appetite. It should show some improvement in the next few days.

The family doctor visit went well also. He examined Judy, assessing for aspects of general health. He commented that she looked much better than the last time he saw her. Of course the last time he saw her, she was still in the hospital following that frightening episode of adverse effects related to the steroid administration. Just about anything would be an improvement when compared to that incident.

Now for the vacation update. We did make it to our planned reunion in Alabama. We traveled on the light side—as far as daily mileage—this was less stressful for Judy and we made reasonable progress.

We had a great time visiting with all our friends, seeing the sights, and making the most of our time in the South. We enjoyed a dinner play that was not only entertaining, but educational as well.

We got to see some of the workings of the TVA (Tennessee Valley Authority) around the area where the reunion was held. Some folks toured a Civil War battlefield, while others, including Judy and I, opted to tour the Unclaimed Baggage Center in Scottsboro.

Of course, I must admit that we all did what we do best at these events—EAT. We sampled the full gamut—from bratwurst to catfish and just about everything in between. We also had a wine tasting of sorts that included genuine Mosel wine—direct from Germany. That brought back memories!

The game of choice this time around turned out to be a bean bag game with wooden ramps with a target hole at the top. This game drew on Judy's former bowling skillset and brought her keen sense of competition to the forefront; she loved it. Folks practiced and honed their skills whenever they had a chance. On the last day, we held a couples' tournament, competing by states. It was a hard-fought single elimination competition. In the end, Judy and I were fortunate to win the "traveling trophies." We now get to display them—at least until the next reunion which is scheduled for three years from now in Minnesota.

We had a great time and although it tested Judy's limits, this was one of the goals that she was determined to accomplish—and she came through with flying colors.

Having proven to ourselves that we are able to deal with the logistics and realities of travel—as the current situation now dictates—we are encouraged and confident that we will be able to complete more of our travel plans in the future.

As always, we thank all of you for keeping us in your hearts and prayers. We would ask that you also pray for all the others who are fighting this terrible affliction.

Earle & Judy

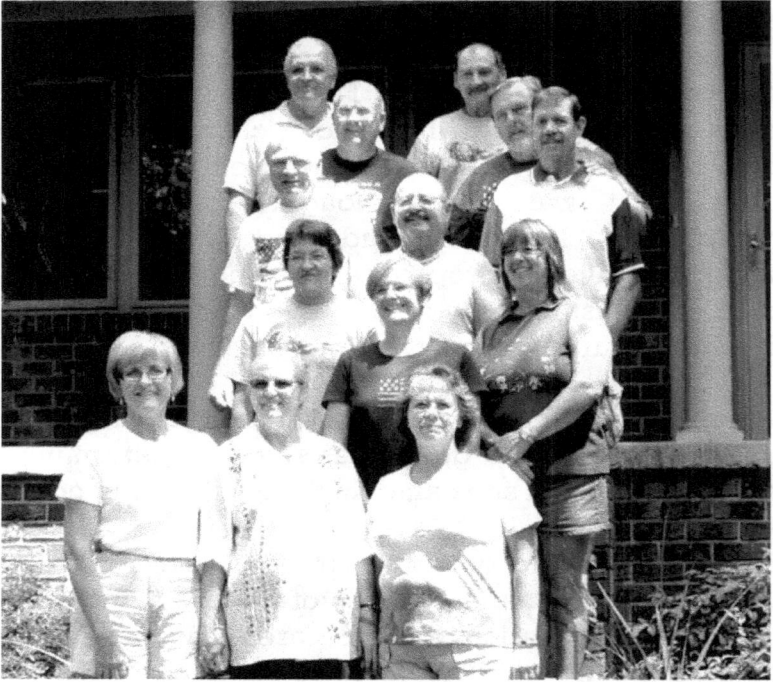

Judy and Earle with some of their "Hahn family" at the 2010 reunion in Alabama.

In this update, we share what we took as disappointing, but not completely unexpected news. We also receive—what at the time, we took to be incidental—news of increased activity of the tumors.

This news would turn out to be the most important turn of events to take place in the recent history of Judy's battle with Inflammatory Breast Cancer and its many complications. We did not recognize it as such at the time, but our journey was about to take another detour.

Wednesday, July 21, 2010

There have been some new events recently, so we now have a couple of days to catch up on. On Tuesday the 20th, we saw the gastrointestinal specialist and learned that at this time, Judy's physical condition and the current regimen of chemotherapy make it a virtual impossibility to perform a reversal of the emergency surgery that saved Judy's life a little over a year ago. This was the "temporary" colostomy necessitated by the bowel rupture. (*In cases where the damaged intestines have healed sufficiently, a reattachment of the bowel ends—called anastomosis—can be performed. This reestablishes normal body function, thereby eliminating the need for a colostomy.*) Dr. G. said that this does not mean that we will never be able to affect the reversal, but that it is simply not a viable option at this time.

As you can imagine, we were disappointed to get the official decision, but since we were aware of this possibility, we were not taken completely off guard with the announcement. As you can probably also understand, the colostomy governed many aspects of our lives—from the briefest of outings to extended travel. Its challenges necessitated many lifestyle adjustments for both of us to consider at every turn.

Today, we saw the radiologist. His news was both encouraging and a little surprising. He was pleased with Judy's overall condition and her amazing continued ability to bounce back from all of the treatments and procedures which she has recently endured. She passed his Q&A and the quick physical checkup with flying colors. However, he did inform us that the latest MRI showed some unexpected activity and new spots of possible cancer.

Since Judy is otherwise healthy and not experiencing any symptoms at present, it was the general agreement of all of the doctors to keep a close eye on the situation and reevaluate with a short-term MRI in eight weeks. Future decisions on a course of action will be based on what they learn from that test. We are cleared to continue the rest of our scheduled summer activities and are looking forward to completing the remainder of our plans.

As always, we extend our thanks to everyone for their continued support, thoughts, and prayers. We truly draw strength from all of your encouragement. Thank you, one and all.

Earle & Judy

The primary focus of the next message is to explain the longer-than-normal gap between updates. Some sort of "bug" had again infected our computers.

Monday, August 16, 2010

This will be just a quick note to let you all know that we are fine. Our computers have been down for a few days. They have just been returned to Operational

Status this evening. I will send a current update in the near future.

Best to all.

Earle & Judy

In this update, I took the liberty to vent about our internet provider. I am reluctant to embrace change—of any sort—as will be readily apparent. There were the looming technical difficulties that cropped up and had to be dealt with before regular updates could begin again.

Later in the note, we share the ongoing concern of all of the doctors about the increasing activity that is showing up in the tests. In retrospect, we did not give these signs the attention they should have commanded. We were riding high on the gains and improvements of the past few months.

Monday, September 20, 2010

Before we get into the update, I need to point out that since a major computer problem occurred and was compounded by the subsequent actions of my Cyber-Nazi internet provider, I no longer have use of the *IncreadiMail* program which we had utilized in the past. Due to the obstacle this has presented, all of my contact information and the ability to form contact groups as done previously, has been hindered. I can only hope that I am able to send this to all my former recipients.

Now, the update: we saw the radiologist today to get the latest MRI reading. He was cagey—to say the least—in the way he answered our questions. He did state that the area of concern has shown some activity. It is, in fact, a little larger than before, but not so much as to warrant any immediate actions. He did, however, tell us that he wants us to set up an appointment with the neurosurgeon, Dr. J. At that time, he (Dr. J.) will be the decision-maker as to when, or whether or not, they will need to intercede surgically.

Although we received no firm answers, we are not jumping to any conclusions. We will hold off making any decisions until we speak with Dr. J.

We hope this finds all of you well. We are ever grateful for all your support, wishes, and prayers.

Earle & Judy

Again, a longer than normal time has elapsed since the last update. Numerous things have been happening, but at such a swift pace that reporting them became secondary for a while.

The rapid-fire changes, coupled with the fact that this was the normally busy season for me at work, combined to interrupt the regular flow of information regarding Judy's state. The conditions of Judy's ailment were changing, but we were devoid of the ability to recognize the importance of the facts because they had presented themselves in such quick succession.

We were still in that euphoric state of mind where everything was going well and our medical team had everything under control. The recent improvements in Judy's condition were encouraging beyond description.

To be confronted with the harsh reality that they were about to amount to naught was not within our ability to grasp at this juncture. We were in for a rude awakening.

Wednesday, November 3, 2010

We had the much-anticipated meeting with the neurosurgeon today. He had a mixed bag of information for us. For the most part, it was better than we expected.

From the last MRI which was completed in September, he tells us that there are four areas of concern. Two are unchanged; one is smaller than previously noted; the last is indeterminately different. The questionable spot could be the result of the radiation and the subsequent necrosis of the irradiated tumor (*a mass of dead tissue cells is referred to as necrosis*). At this point, he sees no reason for any changes to the current treatment and wants to do a follow-up MRI in December.

In the testing arena, Judy is scheduled for a bone scan and a CT scan next Monday to be certain that there are no other areas of concern. She is scheduled to meet with the oncologist the following week. At that time, he should have the results of those tests.

Judy's Journey

Most recently, Judy has been experiencing some increased problems with balance and memory. The general consensus is that these are the aftereffects of the radiation and the cumulative effects of the current chemotherapy treatments. These side effects are disruptive, but not debilitating. We are able to deal with them by taking additional precautions and writing things down.

Judy is now using a cane for increased stability when walking. In general, she is doing as well as can be expected. Her spirit and strength continue to inspire me.

We thank each of you for keeping us in your hearts and prayers and wish the best to all of you for Thanksgiving. We certainly have much to be thankful for.

Earle & Judy

On the surface, the situation seems to be getting more serious as the days pass. The reality is that we are only seeing the tip of the proverbial iceberg. Blissfully unaware, we have been making plans for eventualities —that are never to be.

Once again, we are on that roller coaster of hope, only to be slammed with another harsh reality at the very next turn. In retrospect, it was at about this time that our medical team started to hint a bit more overtly at the severity and lethalness of Judy's condition. We were still not ready to hear what they were saying.

Tuesday, November 16, 2010

Today, we had the eagerly anticipated meeting with the radiologist to get the bone scan and the CT scan results, as well as the all-important findings of the most recent MRI. The first tests show no advancement of the cancer anywhere throughout her body or bones. This, in itself, is good news. This confirms for us that the procedures we are following are working. They are protecting Judy from the all-too-common spread of the disease—metastasis: the dreaded invasion of a primary cancer to other sites in the body.

At this juncture, what we are most interested in is the MRI interpretation. For some time, we have been aware of Judy's increasing frailty and worsening symptoms. Her balance continues to deteriorate. Her cognitive abilities: long term memory, the ability to retain a train of thought, and her immediate recall have all been showing signs of increasing decline.

We were prepared for some bad news from this MRI reading. What we got was a combination of bad news and good news. The bad news was not as bad as we had prepared ourselves for; the good news was better than we could have hoped.

The bad news was: there is, in fact, activity in the tumors throughout her head. Some of the areas may well be the result of the scar tissue surrounding the tumor, but other sites are of greater concern. There is a cluster of small tumors in the back of her neck in the region called the cerebellum. *(The cerebellum is that part of the brain responsible for maintaining balance,*

243

body posture, and equilibrium; coordinating motor movement; steadiness of gait while walking; synchronizing the timing and force of actions; and maintaining muscle tone. It is also involved in some language-related functions.)

Everyone who has read the MRI tends to agree that this tumor activity is responsible for most of the problems which Judy has been experiencing. This area has been irradiated twice now. The radiologist is more than "somewhat reluctant" to recommend additional radiation because of the potential long-term, possibly permanent, side effects that would likely result. He explained that the location of the tumor cluster does open up the potential option of surgically removing them. He was concerned as to how we would react to the recommendation of additional surgery. In truth, we were encouraged that he was able to suggest an active option to pursue. We assured him that, given the current situation, another surgery was not something we were apprehensive about—especially since it would be Dr. J. who will be doing the surgery. He is the neurosurgeon who has performed two brain surgeries on Judy already. We jokingly say that "he has a long history of being inside Judy's head." All kidding aside, we have the utmost faith and trust in his abilities.

(Later...)
I was unable to finish this update on the 16th. It is now Wednesday morning as I try to wrap up. We have finally heard from Dr. J.'s office. We are scheduled for our pre-op consultation with him this afternoon at 3:30. We interpret this to mean that there will probably not be a long delay between the decision to operate and

the actual event. There will be more to follow as this latest plot twist develops.

As we have repeatedly mentioned throughout this entire odyssey, thank you, each and every one of you, for your continued support, heartfelt encouragement, and prayers. Whether you know it or not, each of you has been an integral part of our ongoing battle. You have championed Judy's continued resilience—in what can only be described as a monumental display of will and determination—to overcome the horrific disease she is facing. She is doing so with strength and dignity.

Once again—Thank You for your support.

Earle & Judy

As the end of the year and the combined holidays approach, the situation is changing. The wheels are turning faster and faster, as the roller coaster begins traveling out of control. The transformation is occurring much more rapidly than we can imagine possible.

Though the doctors continue to extend hope and the possibility of new or different treatments, mixed messages are beginning to creep into the consultations. The reality is just starting to set in. We attempt to present a positive outlook to our still-increasing list of update recipients, but the seriousness of the advancing disease is difficult to mask.

Judy's Journey

Wednesday, November 17, 2010

We met with Dr. J., the neurosurgeon, today. At this time, he is not comfortable with recommending the surgery which we discussed earlier with the radiologist. He maintains that the difference in the tumor at this time is only of concern because it has increased in size in spite of the extended continuation of the chemotherapy treatment protocol.

The resulting plan is to repeat the tests again in January as long as the symptoms do not become more intense. At that time, we will see if there is sufficient reason to reconsider the surgical option. We are both comfortable with this proposal. We will continue to monitor Judy's symptoms and wait it out to see what happens in January.

Thanks again for all your continued support.

Earle & Judy

Nearly two weeks later, the oncologist steps in and makes a dramatic change in the treatment plan. Since the tumors do not seem to be responding to the current medication, he opts to try a different form of oral chemotherapy.

This should have set off warning bells, but we completely trusted that the doctors were able to handle the situation. We continued to live in a state of denial.

At this point, Judy had withstood many crises in this battle that she had been so valiantly waging. She had already faced—and overcome—so many challenges; we had every confidence in her ability to conquer this latest attack on her well-being.

Monday, November 29, 2010

Following Judy's recent tests and MRI, her oncologist determined to make a change in the course of treatment we have been following. The last few months of the Tykerb and Xeloda treatment have been disappointing to all of us. In spite of the uninterrupted chemotherapy drugs being administered, the tumors continued to grow. This was definitely not the desired result. As of this past Saturday, we have started a new treatment course with Temodal. (*Google* it if you would like to know more.) The initial dose was not handled well. One of the side effects is nausea and Judy was seriously affected with this undesirable nuisance. Saturday was definitely not a good day. After reviewing the informational insert that came with the meds, I contacted the on-call doctor at her treatment center. It was determined that she should have also been prescribed an anti-nausea medication to be taken a half hour prior to taking the new pills. Sunday and Monday were much better, once we began the co-administration of the Zofran (the nausea preventive medication) along with the Temodal. Zofran is apparently highly effective for managing severe nausea. It has made the new treatment much more tolerable. Hopefully, this new chemotherapy drug will have the desired effect of suppressing the tumors. In January, we should find out when the next MRI will be scheduled.

In the meantime, Judy's balance and cognitive skills are still impaired, but both her will and spirit remain strong. She is still able to manage her bird feeders and keep her fish tanks maintained. She tires easily, but is always ready to tackle whatever needs to be done. When I am asked about her condition, I always tell folks that "she is holding her own," as indeed she is.

We are most thankful for all of you and the generous way you have kept us in your hearts and prayers. Thank you once again.

We hope everyone had an enjoyable Thanksgiving and are now set for the upcoming holidays.

Earle & Judy

Two weeks have passed. In the interim, I have officially retired and am now better able to care for Judy's needs on a daily basis. Now, I am also available to accompany her to the increasing number of appointments which have been scheduled.

We continue to adapt to the perpetually changing conditions of Judy's illness and to the associated circumstances related to it. With alarm, we both realize that the situation is becoming increasingly dire. In addition to the advancing symptoms, the doctors are starting to send mixed messages. One is discouraged by the progress, while another is upbeat and encouraging. We, of course, choose to align ourselves with the latter.

Tuesday, December 14, 2010

We hope that you are all getting into the holiday spirit and rejoicing in the season. We haven't had our first snow yet, so we are still waiting for that final touch to set the mood.

In the past few days, we have met with the oncologist and the radiologist. The oncologist was primarily interested in how Judy was tolerating the new chemotherapy regimen. We related the initial difficulties with nausea and vomiting, but assured him that we were coping much better now. The new procedure is markedly different from the one it replaced and it took a little getting used to. He questioned us about the presenting symptoms of concern: balance, memory, appetite, and such. He has arranged for us to return after the second round of the new pills.

Apparently, they have to continually assess for various side effects, as well as any adverse events while she is taking these substances. We noticed that he was not as upbeat as he usually is. His more restrained mood seemed to communicate itself to us as well; we left the appointment feeling a little down.

Today, we met with the radiologist and he was much more positive. His primary concern was focused on the continuing headaches. He is arranging for an MRI after the first of the year and will be consulting with the neurosurgeon after the results are available. The underlying question is whether or not another surgery would be beneficial. He indicated that the normal treatment at this point would be a form of steroids, but given Judy's past inability to tolerate them, we favor exploring alternative options first. We left his office with a more optimistic outlook. Having a direction and a plan in place usually generates a sense of optimism for both Judy and I.

As the days progress, Judy's outward symptoms continue to intensify. She has increased problems with her balance, stamina, short-term memory, and cognitive agility. The headaches have become more frequent and more debilitating. The doctor has assured us that if the current medications fail to remediate them, we have many rungs left on the ladder of pain management. The one thing that remains unchanged is Judy's strong spirit and determined will.

The continued support provided by of all of you, as well as your prayers and the fact that she knows you are all in her corner give her—I should say, give us—the strength to forge onward. Thank you for your generous and caring support.

We both wish you all a Merry Christmas and a Happy and Prosperous New Year.

Earle & Judy

Just over a week later, two days before Christmas, another hurdle emerges to challenge Judy's well-being. This time the signs are ominous and overwhelmingly clear to others. We are so close to the situation that we "cannot see the forest" for the proverbial trees. I continue to deny the obvious. Somehow, we cannot accept what has become increasingly apparent to those around us—the disease is gaining the upper hand.

Once again, the quick response on the part of the medical staff staves off the short-term crisis, but the long-term outlook is becoming more and more discouraging. In spite of everything, Judy continues to tenaciously fight the monster that is forcibly taking her away from us.

The message begins with well wishes to our on-line family and friends. The tone of our cheery holiday greeting is immediately tempered by our grim report.

Thursday, December 23, 2010

We hope you and all of those close to you are prepared and ready to share in the special time that is upon us. We wish you all a Merry Christmas and a most Happy New Year.

Our holiday plans took a dramatic turn today. Judy has been struggling for the past two or three days. We have concluded that this was probably due to the increased activity of last-minute Christmas shopping. Today, she had a doctor's appointment which was a follow-up to evaluate her response to the latest chemotherapy treatment.

While getting ready to leave the house, Judy was despondent. She was unable to get up without assistance and could not seem to manage to walk on her own. I got the walker out, thinking that it would help her get around, but she was unable to figure out how to use it. I provided step-by-step coaching: first directing her to move her foot, then to move the walker. There simply seemed to be no comprehension—she just stood there. When I said again "move your foot forward," her response was "I don't know what you mean." There are no words which could sufficiently express my feelings of utter helplessness at that moment.

After much effort, we made it to the appointment. While having her labs drawn, she continued to be groggy and lethargic and was unable to participate in the procedures. It was determined that her white blood count was low, her blood pressure was low, and that she was dehydrated. They immediately transfused a liter of saline into her port to rehydrate her. The doctor also decided to give her a small dose of steroids to reduce any swelling that might be compromising her brain function. While the fluids were being infused intravenously, it was determined that it would be necessary to admit her to the hospital in order to increase her stamina.

The MRI that was to have been done in January would be done now to further assist in assessing her condition. At this time, the oncologist indicated that he thought the tumor was continuing to grow in spite of the chemotherapy currently being delivered. He also indicated that the chemo drug that he was administering was the final weapon in his arsenal of chemical agents—he had no additional procedures to offer Judy.

The bottom line was that if the MRI showed further growth, our last hope for relief would lie with the neurosurgeon. At this point, Judy has had the MRI and we are awaiting its reading and interpretation.

The next step will be for the neurosurgeon to evaluate it and determine whether or not surgery will offer any hope for the situation which now appears to be quite desperate.

Judy is in the hospital at present. When I saw her last, she was being set up for additional fluids, as well as platelets to help restore her levels closer to normal. No long-term course of action has been determined yet. The focus is to get her stabilized and to work on her stamina and balance problems.

At this juncture, it would appear that she will be in the hospital through the holidays. Any decision about discharge will be deferred until her condition improves.

Judy has rallied repeatedly in the face of overwhelming odds. Let us pray that she can summon the strength and determination to do so once more. For those in the immediate area, she is in the hospital—Room (omitted),

Judy's Journey

Bed #2. She is able to receive phone calls and short personal visits should anyone wish to stop by.

Now, more than ever in the course of her treatment, she could use your prayers. Thank you in advance for your collective prayers, heartfelt best wishes, and support.

Best wishes to all for the holidays. We wish you all a Merry Christmas and Happy New Year.

Earle

Due to the overwhelming number of update recipients combined in the address books of both Judy's and my computers, we had adopted a system whereby I would pen the original message, usually with Judy's input and approval, then send it out to my list of contacts—which included Judy. She would then forward the message to those on her list of contacts. In this manner, her communications would appear to have come directly from her. Her contacts would often reply directly to her. Due to Judy's weakened condition and the seriousness of the current situation, I had to change the rules of the game.

At this time, I advised her friends and acquaintances that things were not as they appeared to be. Although they were still getting a message from Judy's email address, it was being sent by me. I also informed them that Judy would be unable to respond to any of their replies at this time.

A hospital stay at Christmas would be discouraging to anyone, but at this juncture, it was also a major wake-up call for all of us. Then, once again, to everyone's amazement, the situation appeared to have been brought under control with the administration of some relatively simple medical procedures. For Judy, it was another obstacle faced and overcome; or so it would seem.

Friday, December 24, 2010

Everybody, please note that I (Earle) am sending this out via Judy's e-mail. She is not sending it, nor is she able to respond to any of your replies. She is still in the hospital. Managing the computer is beyond her current ability at this stage of her recovery. Thanks.

EW

Merry Christmas All!

"What a difference a day makes!" How many times have we heard that phrase? I can tell you from firsthand experience that, once again, a single day has surely made an immense difference.

During the day to which I allude—today—Judy has had IV fluids, two pints of blood, and has started a regimen of low dose steroids. The difference which these interventions have made is nothing short of amazing. Judy is much more alert. She is able to participate in her care and is already showing signs of strength and coordination which were not imagined possible, just yesterday.

Today's theory is that the combination of dehydration, deconditioning, and increased pressure from the tumor were responsible for yesterday's state of confusion and inability to coordinate thought, function, and physical action. The MRI has shown a "slight"—and the emphasis is on "slight"—increase in the one tumor that they have continued to monitor closely. This change is still thought to be a result of increased necrosis (dead tissue cell debris) caused by the tumor being targeted and destroyed by the radiation treatment.

We will meet with the neurosurgeon tomorrow, but having met with his P.A. today, that seems to be the best theory to date.

The biggest culprit in this latest episode appears to be the dehydration factor. How many times have we heard about the dangers of dehydration? It has been a topic of discussion between ourselves and the doctors—all of the doctors—many times.

This event dramatically supports every warning which we have ever heard about the seriousness of this condition. Following the administration of a single liter of IV fluids, the improvement was immediately noticeable.

In light of this, Judy and I have discussed how best to remediate the problem of her not drinking enough water. I have found one particular flavored-water which does not use artificial sweetener. Judy has tried it and is agreeable to using it in order to increase her intake of fluids.

Judy's blood counts were low. The white count is low due to a side effect of her most recent chemotherapy treatment. Her red count was apparently down for a variety of reasons, but two pints of whole blood remedied that deficiency.

The decision to start the steroids was a difficult one to make. Her past experience with that treatment has left us all cautious about using them again. Due to the gravity of the situation, it was decided to start a low dose regimen and closely monitor her reaction. So far, the combined protocols have yielded a marked improvement. While Judy admittedly still has more ground to cover, today's proposal of initiating physical therapy tomorrow is a major step toward a recovery that many doubted possible yesterday.

Once again, she has found the strength, resilience, and courage to rally when all the odds seemed impossibly stacked against her. While we certainly give credit to the doctors and the medical staff working with Judy, I know that your continued support and prayers have played a big part in her turnaround. Thank you, to each and every one, for that unwavering support.

Merry Christmas and Happy New Year to you all!

Earle

Christmas was brightened by the continued improvement Judy was exhibiting in the hospital. The next three days' updates were increasingly upbeat and positive, raising everyone's hopes that we were on the road to recovery once again. Unbeknown to us, in reality, what we were on was the last incline on that never-ending roller coaster on which we had been riding for more than two and a half years.

Saturday, December 25, 2010 Christmas Day

We hope that you all had a Merry Christmas and enjoyed the special day with your family and loved ones.

(Sorry this wasn't sent first thing this morning, but unfortunately, my computer took a "hissy fit" at about 0300 hours and deleted everything except the first line which you see above. I was so upset that I wanted to inflict pain on the computer. I, instead, opted to set it aside and come back this morning with a clearer mind.)

This report is as of 12/25...

We saw the neurosurgeon in the morning. He confirmed his P.A.'s diagnosis: the tumor that is of primary concern—there are three, but this is the only one that appears active—shows a minimal increase in size at this time. It has gone from "1.9 to 2.2" in whatever metric measurement they deal in, millimeters, I believe. *(To put this in perspective—there are 2 ½ centimeters in an inch. Since a millimeter is one tenth of a centimeter, one inch would equal 25 mm. Hence, 2 mm would be a little less than 1/10th of an inch).* At any rate, the neurosurgeon does not believe this actually represents tumor growth. He believes that it is more likely the cellular fragments of the dead—or dying—

tumor; the result of the radiation treatments. This being the case, he does not think that the tumor growth was responsible for this recent episode.

With that resolved, we can concentrate on the more mundane causes of the situation that resulted in Judy's admission to the hospital.

Primarily, dehydration proved to be the main underlying problem. This, in concert with the physical deconditioning—the complication resulting from sleeping 16 to 18 hours a day—caused significant disorientation and major confusion. Since the administration of the saline and two pints of whole blood, she has been much more lucid.

We have discussed this problem and have jointly determined a solution. We will substitute flavored water and the sports drinks that she deems tolerable for the plain water, which she genuinely dislikes. We are working our way through the available products now.

I anticipate that a physical therapist will probably start working with her soon. Some additional therapy (or possibly even rehab) will probably also be initiated in the near future. All of these possibilities are tremendously less complicated now that I am retired and available for chauffeur duties 24/7.

Judy has been showing improvement, even if only slight, as each day goes by. We are not pressuring the nurses or doctors about a release date. We are depending on their judgment as to when she is adequately recovered to safely return home.

Judy's Journey

Again, we hope you all had a Merry Christmas. Later, I will attempt to attach a picture of Judy wishing you all just that! We join together in thanking you for your much appreciated support and prayers.

Earle

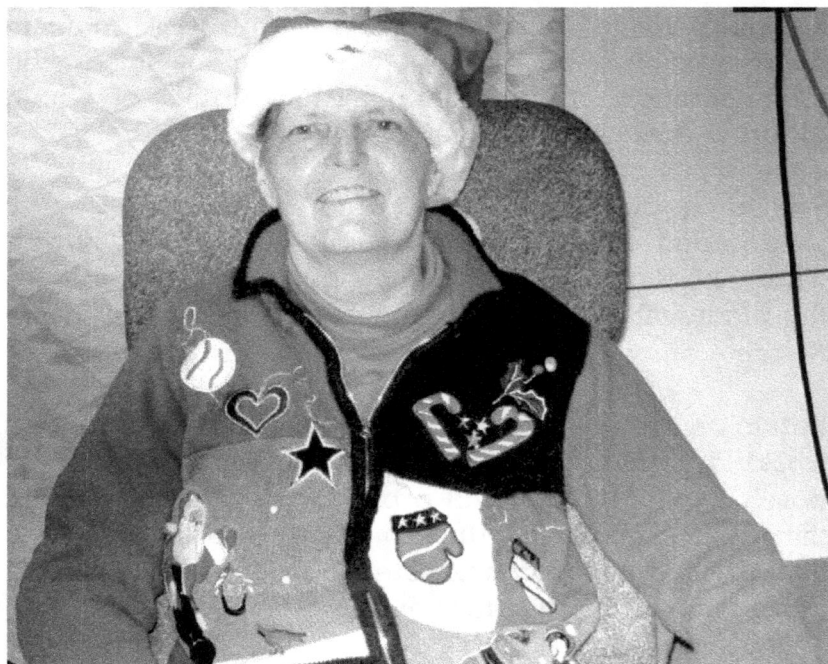

Christmas 2010 ~ No matter how she felt,
Judy always had a smile to share.

Sunday, December 26, 2010

While the current situation exists, I plan to continue providing daily updates. The length will depend upon how much news there is to impart. The updates will be short when the information to be shared is minimal. I expect today's report to be brief.

I spent a good portion of the day in preparation for the promised storm in our forecast. I made it to the hospital with the day's samples of flavored water and sports drinks about 1:00 p.m. Judy was just finishing lunch. Her appetite is still alarmingly slight, but when I asked why she was not getting the appetite enhancer she was taking at home, I was told that the steroids she was now receiving were expected to resolve that. We are still waiting on that point.

When I am in the room, I take it upon myself to perform any of the staff functions which I am comfortable doing. Since they made the mistake of showing me how to disarm the bed alarm, my list of "capabilities" is growing. Tonight, while helping Judy with one of the frequent bathroom calls, Judy was not only able to pull herself up out of the bed, but at one point, she stood unaided and remained reasonably steady for several seconds.

These are small milestones indeed, but certainly measurable steps in the right direction. When I inquired, the nurse said that it would be reasonable to expect the PT team to start working with her this week. I hope to be able to report on more noticeable gains when they start.

The weekend brought Judy many visitors, all enjoyable, but none as memorable as that of our great-granddaughter, Jaidyn. She, of course, steals the show and the hearts of everyone who meets her. Being able to spend some time with her lifts Judy's spirits so much! Our daughter, Chris came home from her vacation in sunny Florida. She is Jaidyn's grandmother and I enjoy reminding her at every opportunity that she is "<u>Grammy</u> Chris" now—it's <u>my</u> turn to tease! She made it in just ahead of the storm and came up to visit. That gave Judy another boost to her spirits.

In closing, we of course thank everyone for their support and prayers.

Earle

As an after-thought, in case you do not have firsthand experience with the effects of dehydration, *Google*: "Adult Dehydration Symptoms"—it is quite educational.

E

Monday, December 27, 2010

Short and sweet tonight—the doctor was in this morning, assessed Judy and noted the improvement in her condition. He then asked the magic question "Are you ready to go home?" Well, I suppose you can guess her answer. He arranged for one test—a spine MRI. He informed her that if that looked good and she would agree to go to physical therapy to build up her lower body strength, he would discharge her. At this point, her departure is only penciled in, but steps are already underway to get her home.

The discharge planner came by to talk with us and has already set up a PT appointment with the folks here in town. It would appear that we are really on the road home and just need the doc to give the nod to "make it so." (Any "Trekkies" out there should recognize this one.) When this actually happens, I will let everyone know just as soon as we are settled in. We would certainly not want the folks in the area to be visiting strangers in Judy's old room at the hospital.

If we are able to bring her home tomorrow, it will undoubtedly be due to the combined efforts of Judy's indomitable will and strength, the excellent care that she received at the hospital, and perhaps most of all, the power of all of you and your combined prayers and support. I am without the words to convey my deepest thanks to all of you. It doesn't seem like enough, but nevertheless, thank you, one and all.

As an aside; our blizzard was a bust. We picked up about six inches of snow, but the winds, with gusts of 50 mph or so, have been, and continue to be, incredible. The snow totals were far short of the predicted amounts, but sufficient to get us into the winter mindset. Now we can start thinking of spring and the day when Pitchers and Catchers are to report.

Thanks again!

Earle

Judy's Journey

Following several days of seemingly-encouraging progress, the day we all knew would arrive, did in fact, do just that.

We had reached the top of the "virtual" roller coaster ride. The final frightening descent was about to commence. While relentlessly clinging to some degree of hope, it was time to face reality. The reality was harsh, formidable, and difficult to accept.

Dr. K., the radiologist, delivered the news. I have often wondered how he came to be the messenger. Perhaps it was because he was the newest addition to the team of specialists who had been treating Judy. For whatever reason, he apparently drew the short straw and became the emissary who would deliver the devastating announcement. The normally upbeat Dr. K. was visibly shaken that day.

Tuesday, December 28, 2010

I have been putting this off for as long as I can. This update will not be an easy one to write, edit, or send.

Our radiologist, Dr. K., came by to see us this afternoon. It seems that those whom I have long-dubbed the "Three Amigos"—the oncologist, the radiologist, and the neurosurgeon—have been in somber consultation with each other several times this week. In fact, they had two face-to-face meetings today alone, a rare event indeed. The goal of their efforts was to redefine Judy's current condition, examine and explore the options, reach a definitive conclusion, and finally, to formulate recommendations as to how to proceed.

The oncologist indicated that he has exhausted all of the medical and chemotherapy options for her treatment. The last two chemo treatments did not produce the desired effect and, in fact, the tumors continued to increase in size during the administration of the chemotherapy agents. This was definitely not a good outcome. Regretfully, he informed us that he has expended his last viable option.

The radiologist stated his case succinctly: Judy has had massive amounts of radiation in both "whole brain" and focused protocols. To subject her to further radiation would almost certainly produce negative consequences to her very being. There would be no assurance that additional treatments would yield any positive results at this stage of the disease process.

The oncologist and radiologist both turned to the neurosurgeon as their absolute final hope. Before making a decision, they pulled all of the MRIs which detailed the progression of the tumors. After careful study, they all agreed that the changes displayed were due to active tumor cells and not merely to necrosis, as had been previously hoped. It was further noted that the only logical surgery that could be considered would involve the removal of all three of the identified tumors.

Dr. J., the neurosurgeon declared emphatically: it was his carefully considered opinion that Judy was not strong enough to survive the surgery. If by some remote possibility she did, there was a good chance that there would be irreparable damage and that major complications would likely result. Of greatest significance, there was a potentially high risk for major personality changes.

Dr. K. affirmed that they all think the world of Judy and want only what is best for her. They have come to think of her as being as close as a family member. They do not want to see her suffer, nor do they wish her general well-being further compromised. With this in mind, they have reached the painful conclusion—all that can be done has been done.

They somberly recommend that we plan for the inevitable while we are both still able to make clear decisions. Their goal now is to manage the current debilitating symptoms and get Judy strong enough to return home. They have outlined the options available to us: the Visiting Nurse Association, Hospice Services, and other organizations which become resources at times such as these.

As much of a shock and bewildering disappointment as this meeting was, our doctors have done for us exactly what we asked them to do at the start of this odyssey. We asked them not to talk to us in veiled references and innuendos, but rather to tell us the truth straight out so that we can deal with it. Judy and I did not want to be caught unaware, particularly as significant changes became imminent.

In spite of how difficult this devastating declaration is for us to accept, they have ultimately been faithful in honoring our request. For respecting that trust and for all their valiant efforts, we are truly grateful.

Judy and I have had an initial discussion about how to proceed. For now, we have decided to put first things first—that is to get her home and to keep her at home for as long as possible. We have known this day was coming from the beginning, but we had hoped that its arrival would not have occurred so soon. We will, however, face this like we have everything over the years—together.

From the bottom of our hearts, we thank everyone who has been beside us, with us, and behind us throughout this journey. Know in your hearts that your support has meant much to both of us. We are, and will be, eternally grateful for your support. We will, in whatever future remains, keep you all informed as to whatever progress is made.

Thank you again for your wishes and prayers.

Earle

Tuesday, December 28, 2010

A quick note –

For anyone who has *"Semper Fi"* in their background, remember the motto: "Adapt, Adapt, Adapt." This is what we are doing.

I was at the hospital this morning when the doctor came by. At first, I wasn't sure she was a doctor as she looked more like a *Miss America* contestant, but she was indeed the doc—one of those "hospitalists." She informed us that the spine MRI came back clean; some arthritis, but no growths (tumors).

This, and the fact that they are pleased with her recovery to this point, was the good news. The less than good news is that Judy has developed a urinary tract infection and they want to get that under control before releasing her. This seems perfectly logical and prudent to both of us, a little disappointing, but the right thing to do. We will take it one day at time until the infection has abated.

Judy will be staying in the hospital for at least one more day and we will see how things progress tomorrow.

As always, thank you for your concern, best wishes, and your heartfelt prayers.

Earle

As 2010 comes to a close, we get a slight reprieve. Judy's condition improves sufficiently to permit a discharge from the hospital and make the trip home. Of course, there are more hurdles to overcome, but we have been in this fight for a long time and don't expect to face anything we can't handle together.

The update concludes with the two of us back home, settled in, and ready to face whatever fate has in store for us. We are appreciative of every blessing that has come our way including the priceless comfort we draw from the knowledge that we are home and together. At this moment, nothing else matters.

Wednesday, December 29, 2010

Today brought an unexpected blessing. Judy called me after the doctor made rounds this morning, to let me know that she was being discharged. This, of course, was the news we were waiting for, but experience has taught us "not to count our chickens before they are hatched," so we were hesitant to hope or plan too much in advance. When I got to the hospital with most of the things needed for going home, I found the changes and Judy's improvement from the day before simply amazing. The antibiotics had already taken effect. The UTI that was so bothersome was now all but under control.

Since Chris was joining us at the hospital and was still en route, I pressed her into service to bring the item I forgot at home (did you catch the part where I said that I arrived at the hospital with <u>most</u> of her going home gear?). I forgot her shoes. I plead the 5th.

When all was in place, the paperwork (there's always paperwork) had been completed and lunch served, we got her dressed and headed out. After one stop at the pharmacy, since she has five days of antibiotics yet to finish, we headed for home.

Once there, the first obstacle we faced was the set of four stairs to get into the house. Fortunately, Judy's upper body strength is still remarkable, so I simply got in front of her to support her forward movement. She put her strong foot on the step and while I provided a secure hand-hold, she pulled herself up, one step at a time. Our first challenge had been met and beaten.

Judy's Journey

Once in the house, I offered her the walker, so she could get herself to the living room. With just a little coaching, she was able to maneuver herself right to her favorite chair.

As I write this, we have been home for about six hours. Thus far, we have found a way to overcome everything we have had to face; we have even managed laundry. It all seemed so normal, she giving the orders and me asking dumb questions, but we got it done. We are confident that the move home was the right thing to do—and together—we will be fine.

I have been asked by some folks about coming to see Judy now that she is home. Since I am home now to field the calls, I would just ask that anyone interested in stopping by to visit simply call first. We can then determine what is best, basing any decision on her condition at the time. I expect that she will need a few days to settle in and get caught up on her rest. After that, we will just play it day by day.

As always, thank you for your prayers, support, and the kind, eloquent messages of hope and devotion. We are blessed indeed to have friends and family who have been so supportive. Thanks again.

Earle & Judy

2011

As the New Year starts, we are facing a fresh set of challenges. Some are significantly different from those which we had become accustomed to dealing with in the past. The period immediately following the unforeseen hospital stay presented the most formidable adjustment we had dealt with to date. There were issues of mobility, strength, cognitive impairment, and the ubiquitous dilemma created by Judy's diminished appetite. The one thing that was not missing was Judy's will to fight. Her spirit was strong enough to carry both of us through these difficult days.

The timing of my recent retirement was a major factor in aiding our adjustment to the constantly changing situation. I was able to spend more time with Judy and see to her daily needs. She was no longer facing the everyday obstacles alone. I was now available to ease the myriad of daily trials which she faced due to her diminished capacity to manage many otherwise seemingly-minor challenges. I found it necessary to issue a special notice at the start of this update. I had been handling the outgoing messages to both of our respective email groups, and I don't think I was doing a very good job; hence, the need for a special communication.

Tuesday, January 4, 2011

Special Notice:
This is the first update to go out since I have been able to revise and edit Judy's email group members—with her help, of course. The previous updates went out to group listings that Judy edited just prior to her recent hospital stay. If you are receiving multiples copies of

this message, please let me know and I will correct the listings. If this is the first update which you have received in a long time, contact me at the email address above, let me know the last time you were updated, and I will give you the *Reader's Digest* version of the last two weeks.

Earle

Our recent set of tests and trials are over. Judy has been home from the hospital for almost a week. Now, we are facing the new challenges of being home in what can only be described as a state of recovery—but this is sometimes a veritable "moving target."

The UTI seems to have resolved itself or has now been cleared up by the antibiotics. Either way, it is a welcome step in Judy's recovery. Now, we are concentrating on her regaining strength and increasing her mobility. At this point, her muscle tone and body weakness remain very problematic. The doctors refer to it as a "deconditioned state" which resulted from the dehydration and increased immobility during her recent ailments. Inactivity, as we have so recently discovered, is in itself, debilitating.

Judy is connected with the physical therapy clinic here in town. Yes, I know; anyone familiar with the town of Chester just said "WHERE?" It turns out that there is a top notch PT facility right here in town. The arrangements have already been made for her to receive services there. Judy is involved in a reconditioning program. After only two sessions, she is already showing progress.

Although she is still using the walker to get around, she is displaying better control and agility while moving about. We are confident that our goals of increased independence and mobility are fully attainable. When these targets have been reached, we hope to be able to expand Judy's boundaries and make trips outside of the home for social purposes once again, rather than just medical appointments.

On the topic of the social aspect, for those folks who are interested in visiting Judy, please feel free to call us at the house prior to visiting. It is essential that we first assess her current level of stamina. We can then let you know if it is a good time to stop by or if rescheduling will be necessary. Obviously, some days are still better than others; Judy's recovery must be our first priority.

We thank each of you for your ongoing support and prayers. It is comforting to know that so many people are so supportive and willing to provide whatever level of help they are able to manage. Comforting describes only part of the story; encouraging is probably more accurate. It is only through your support that we have been able to find the strength to persevere in this fight.

Thank you for helping us to find that inner quality so many people have commented on. We really have no idea of what we are capable until we are forced to stretch ourselves, reaching further and deeper than we could ever have imagined. We know that each of you has contributed to that accomplishment.

Earle & Judy

> Less than a week has passed since the last update, but with this next message, we have some positive news to share. Knowing that the update recipients, whom I have now come to think of as "our audience," thrive on good news, I am anxious to impart this information related to Judy's recent progress. The full report is telling as to the severity of the deconditioning that she must overcome, but we are delighted to share what we perceive as such good news. We are actually happy to find ourselves exhausted following such a minor event as going out to breakfast, because it is a step forward. Again, at this point, we still persist in thinking of our current circumstances in terms of a battle that we can win.

Monday, January 10, 2011

Not a lot to report, but good news is always welcome. Regardless of whether it is great or small, to us it is never insignificant.

We've had a busy weekend. Starting on Friday, we had a PT session scheduled in the morning and a last minute doctor's appointment in the afternoon. Judy's PT is progressing well. The gains are in baby steps, but as long as Judy is moving in the right direction, we are happy. I should also mention that her appetite has rebounded as well. I think that as soon as she is able to get around on her own, her first request is going to be to go out to eat. This, as much as I tease her about it, is a good sign and cause for rejoicing. Apparently, certain things are returning to some degree of normalcy.

The doctor's visit went well also. Judy's blood counts have returned to whole numbers and her blood pressure is back in the normal range. They did, however, think it necessary to give her a liter of intravenous fluids. This caused the visit to extend until almost 5:00 p.m., a long day indeed.

Saturday was a quiet day; mostly spent recovering from Friday. Sunday, however, included a first. Sunday morning we made our first foray outside the house for a social, rather than medical destination. We went to Sunday morning breakfast. It is a ritual that we have been following for years, but have not been able to participate in for some weeks.

We had to start early in the morning to meet our old schedule, but it was definitely worth it. We had a great breakfast and enjoyed the visit with my brother, his wife, and our good friends, Frank and Jean. We were home by 8:30 a.m.; it took until almost 1:30 p.m. to recover—but it was very satisfying and certainly worth the effort.

As Judy's strength and stamina return, we are looking forward to seeing all our friends and family who have been so supportive of us during these difficult times.

Judy's Journey

Thanks to everyone for keeping us in your hearts and prayers. We are indeed in your debt. Thank you again.

Earle & Judy

The high spirits from just a week ago have been quickly replaced by new concerns. The ominous ride continues. The peaks are simply a distant memory now as we enter the terrifying troughs. These times are ushered in by way of several intense doctor visits during which we are reintroduced to some now-inarguable facts. The stark reality of our situation has again sprung from the shadows and was staring us right in the face.

This update opens with the words none of us wanted to hear, and that I, for one, found excruciatingly difficult to speak. It was even more heart-wrenching to put down in written words on the page.

The time had come for us to face the certainty of Judy's terminal condition and deal with what we could no longer deny was inevitable. As painful as it was to admit, the demon that we had been battling for almost three years was winning. No amount of human effort could alter the final outcome. It was time for Judy and me to finally admit: all that could be done had been done, and enough was enough.

Judy had fought persistently and valiantly, but her strength was now depleted; her body ravaged by an insidious and tenacious adversary. Exhausted from the struggles required to stay in the fight, she declares that the time has come to allow the disease to run its course—and let be what will be.

Our roller coaster ride was nearing the end; the station was now in sight. We were about to enter a new phase of the journey. Though we had "heard" the ominous prognosis and "accepted" the lack of remaining remedies with our ears, our minds had refused to absorb the dire reality and lethal finality of Judy's condition until now.

As Judy and I traveled this long, arduous road, we have had a personal revelation of the ultimate power of prayer, but even more significantly of the power of the almighty God who hears and answers those prayers. Someone once said that God answers all our prayers, though sometimes his answer is "No." In time, I would also come to understand that there are times when His answer is "Wait" or "I have something better for you." When His answer is "No," the "something better" restores hope for eternal life and wholeness of an immortal body and spirit on the other side.

You know, it's kind of amazing that we, as Christians, hope to spend eternity in Heaven—which is promised to be a better place than that which we know on earth—when we complete our pilgrimage here. Everyone wants to go, but no one wants to die to get there.

"To every thing there is a season, and a time to every purpose under heaven..." (Ecclesiastes 3:1, KJV).

Judy's Journey

Monday, January 17, 2011

"Run its course"

We finally acknowledged that the medical profession had depleted all options and that further treatment of Judy's condition carried a higher percentage of risk than potential benefit. The above statement was the expressed unanimous conclusion of all of us—the doctors, Judy, and I. We now, regretfully, accepted it as being the inevitable.

At the time Judy and I made that decision, we were encouraged by the fact that Judy was able to attain some, albeit limited, mobility. We believed that with PT, she could regain additional freedom of movement and retain a degree of dignity. Our best intentions and plans for the immediate future were not to be.

Judy's condition seemed to be improving with the first few sessions of PT. We were hopeful that this would continue.

In the three days since her last session, things have once again changed dramatically. On Saturday she was noticeably weaker. By Sunday she was unable to find her way to the bathroom and lost the ability to maneuver the course through the house, even with the walker.

As a result of this latest development, we have initiated the process of enrolling her in the VNA program that will most likely start with in-home care and proceed to Home Hospice. This has not been an easy decision to make, but it seems to be the correct one given the circumstances.

Should this turn out to be the way things unfold, there is a strong chance this could be the last update that I send out. I do not intend to detail the final struggles that Judy faces.

I do wish to thank each of you for your unwavering support and encouragement. Your sincere wishes, thoughts, and prayers have all been welcomed and thankfully received.

You have all played a vital role in Judy's battle with this demonic disease. Your support has lifted our spirits in the tough times and has carried us through the dark days. You cannot know how helpful you have all been, and for that, we thank you. Please keep us in your hearts and prayers as we let this affliction ... run its course.

With heartfelt thanks,

Earle & Judy

> This message goes out a mere four days since the last update. We have gone from attending PT sessions in the community to bypassing the expected enrollment in the VNA home care services. Based on the drastically accelerated downward spiral, we have already determined the need to access the Home Hospice division of the organization. This was a major adaptation for us. It required not just physical changes

in and around our home, but a complete modification of our mindsets.

Regretfully, it was time to transition from fighting the disease to simply doing our best to mediate and compensate for the terrible effects of the affliction—during what we now recognized would undoubtedly be Judy's final days—even if only in minute ways.

The rapidity with which the cancer progressed still amazes me today, more than a year after the fact. It was heartbreaking for those of us who had to watch helplessly, as the vibrant woman we knew, as wife, sister, mother, and grandmother slowly faded into a world that we could not know. We could only hope and pray that it would eventually bring her the peace she so richly deserved.

Friday, January 21, 2011

This is just a quick note to let you know how things are going under the new system. We have successfully transitioned into the arena of hospice care. Perhaps, I should say that we are still in the process of transitioning, as I don't think we have met all the folks involved in the program yet.

Our initial visit from the RN and the VNA Hospice Caseworker was on Wednesday. That was a lengthy meeting during which they asked a lot of questions—and I must emphasize *a lot* of questions. They, of course, needed to find out the extent of Judy's situation. They needed to gather all of the relevant information to enable them to provide compassionate, dignified care to Judy at this stage of the disease process, and to help us, the family, as we prepare to let her go. They were here for more than two hours, explaining the program and inquiring about background information. They were quite thorough in their explanation of their role and how the service is managed.

The one thing they both stressed was that their goal is to meet our needs, not to restructure our regimen to meet an arbitrary set of guidelines. They have much to offer and a great deal of flexibility in what they are able to provide. I am comfortable that we made the right decision in signing up for their program.

I would like to cover a couple of things that need to be known by everyone who receives these updates, especially the folks who receive them as a forward in what appears to be a message from Judy. Judy is not, I emphasize **she is not** sending those forwards; I am. She has not had sufficient concentration or coordination to operate her computer for almost two weeks.

If you wish to respond or send a message to Judy, DO NOT send it to her email address. In all likelihood, she will never see it. Instead, please send your replies and messages to me at (email address omitted); I will read your messages to her, just as I am doing with the cards as they arrive.

Also, many friends and family who live in the area have asked about visiting Judy. This is well within the realm of possibility with a few common sense guidelines.

Judy's Journey

First—even though at our last doctor visit her immune system had rebounded to what is considered the low end of normal, she is still quite fragile and should not be exposed to any kind of viruses or infections unnecessarily. If you are not feeling well, please delay your visit until you have completely recovered from your illness.

Second—in all cases, please call ahead to see if she is up to having visitors. Keep in mind that the simple act of trying to be social takes more out of her than we would otherwise expect. Also, please be aware that the person you will be visiting will be vastly different from the Judy you used to know. She has difficulty following a conversation thread; her speech is halting at best. She becomes easily confused or "lost."

Lastly—please keep all of her limitations in mind and don't overtax her stamina and ability to be a good hostess. Please plan to limit your stay to her capacity to withstand the extra demand on her strength. If we keep these guidelines in mind, I am confident that we can accommodate most folks' desire to stop by for some face-to-face time with Judy.

As always, I cannot thank you all enough for your steadfast support and commitment. You are all very dear to us and we thank you for your support, thoughts, and prayers. I really cannot say this enough: Thank You, one and all.

Earle & Judy

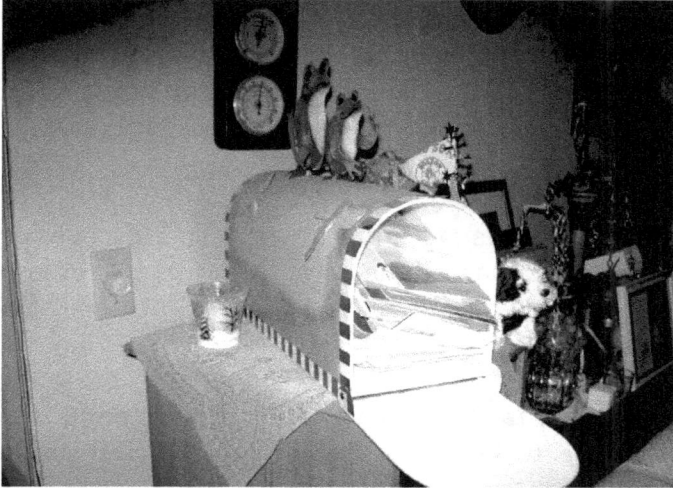

Throughout her valiant battle, Judy received many cards of encouragement—
all of which she saved, enjoying them again and again.

Here, only three days have passed. Already, I find it necessary to modify the plan for visitation that I had so carefully outlined in the last update.

The cancer was raging now and significant changes were occurring on a daily basis. The hospice staff was superb. They provided the rock that I was able to lean on when needed during this incredibly difficult time.

Judy was in and out of awareness and only marginally able to participate in conversation, but when she did, she still managed a jibe or two at my expense. This had long been our pattern and this was how I knew she was really still with us.

Judy's Journey

Monday, January 24, 2011

Judy's condition is deteriorating rapidly. I am sorry to have to do this, but due to changing conditions I no longer have any choice—I must restrict any further physical visits to family only.

Do not take this to mean any drastic change is imminent, just that changes are occurring continually and Judy is less able to handle the added stress of socializing.

If this changes in the future, I will let everyone know. It would be OK to call and if she is up to it, I'll put her on the speaker phone to talk to you.

As always, thank you for your support, caring thoughts, and prayers. We are eternally thankful for all of your encouragement and understanding.

Earle

Five days have passed and I know that our supporters are anxious to hear firsthand news as to how the situation is unfolding. Sharing honest and up-to-date information with our friends and family was the original goal of the series of updates which now spanned the better part of three years.

As difficult as it was at this juncture, I felt the need to fill the silence with the truth which would carry out that noble purpose and eliminate the speculation that was bound to happen if I let my messages lapse.

Saturday, January 29, 2011

I hope this finds you all well and able to make the most of whatever "Old Man Winter" is bringing you. We have had much in the way of snow, but are holding up.

I feel certain that many of you are anxious to hear of Judy's condition. While I do not wish to go into a lot of details, I will paint a general picture so that you will know the true situation and not have to speculate.

If you remember a few updates back, I outlined our—mostly Judy's—decision to forgo any further treatment and let the condition "run its course." That simple phrase sounded so noble at the time, but it has proven to be overwhelming in its reality. All that can be said is that the process is advancing.

Judy is fully bedridden now. She is sedated most of the time for pain management. She is only minimally able to communicate at this time. There are momentary flashes of cognitive connection, but they are few and far between.

She is under the care of the Home Hospice division of the VNA. We have found them to be wonderful, caring people. Judy's comfort is their primary concern. She is well cared for and someone is by her side at all times.

As difficult as all this is to understand and accept, please know that she is where she wanted to be, home, and surrounded by her loved ones. She is as comfortable as modern medicine is able to make her.

Judy's Journey

All that we ask at this time is that you keep her in your hearts and prayers. Our prayer is that her transition be as gentle as possible into what can only be described as God's plan for us all.

I truly mean it when I say that your support has been vital to sustaining us as we have negotiated the convoluted mazes that have comprised this journey. We have travelled the many peaks of rejoicing and valleys of anguish which have brought us ultimately to this point.

Please accept our heartfelt thanks for all your support, good thoughts, and prayers. Thank you all.

Earle & Judy

Again, just five days have passed since the last update. The message we all knew was coming would now be sent out.

It was a strangely convoluted time, punctuated with a swirl of emotion with which to deal. There was extreme sadness, coupled with an unanticipated feeling of relief. We were saddened to have lost the dearest person in our lives, but simultaneously relieved that she was finally at rest and no longer suffering.

An odd kind of reflexive, almost mechanical, response seemed to have taken over. Everything that needed to be done was accomplished, but I have only the vaguest of memories of what those things were and how they were achieved.

The hospice staff took over and directed most of the official actions. We, the family, had only to attend to the family-related matters.

It was a difficult time, but as the next two updates outline, Judy, who had been our chief managing officer for years, still had a hand in things. All we had to do, one final time, was to follow her instructions.

It should be noted that in the original update which follows, it was mentioned that the calling hours were still pending. In the obituary copy that I have included, all arrangements had been finalized.

Friday, February 4, 2011

Today was the day we all knew was coming but none of us wanted to see arrive.

Judy passed from this world at about noon today. She was where she wanted to be; at home, surrounded by her family. She was under the care of the VNA Hospice staff. She was well cared for and comfortable right to the end. We are all comforted by the fact that she is no longer suffering. She is finally at peace.

I wish to take this, possibly final, opportunity to thank you all for your warm caring thoughts, heartfelt sympathy, and prayers. You have all made this most difficult time an easier burden to bear.

Thank you everyone.

Below, I have included a copy of the obituary submitted to the newspaper. They have been known to edit at will, so I am sending the full version.

The date for the calling hours and the memorial service schedule are not included at this time because we are waiting to hear from an out-of-state family as to their travel plans. When those details have been finalized, I will send them to everyone. The funeral home information is included. Only the dates have been omitted.

Thank you all once again.

Earle

Friday, February 4, 2011 (later in the day)

We have finalized the plans for Judy's memorial service. For anyone who is able to join us, the times and dates follow.

The calling hours will be on Monday, February 7th, from 2:00-4:00 p.m. and 7:00-9:00 p.m. The Memorial Service will be on Tuesday, February 8th, at 11:00 a.m.

For anyone interested in joining the family afterward, there will be a luncheon following. Directions will be announced.

Thank you.

Earle

This is Judy's obituary which appeared in the Union Leader following her demise. Creating the document that would finally go to print, though extremely heart-wrenching and emotional, was actually made a little easier by the fact that Judy—always the pragmatic one—actually helped to compose it in advance of her passing.

In the initial draft, I had made an omission (her first place of employment). Judy immediately picked up on the oversight and had me correct the error and revise the original version.

I like to think that she didn't want to miss that last opportunity to give me instructions. This was a task that she had been shouldering with efficient enthusiasm for in excess of forty years.

Judy L. Whitcher

Chester– Judy L. (Davis) Whitcher, 60, long-time resident of Chester, NH, succumbed after a lengthy battle with breast and brain cancer. She was born in Manchester, on July 31, 1950, the second child of Paul E. and Sylvia L. (Barnes) Davis.

She was a graduate of Manchester Memorial High School and had attended classes at Rivier College in Nashua.

Judy was married at Longmeadow Church in Auburn on March 22, 1969. While her husband served in the USAF, she lived in Las Vegas, Nevada and then spent four years in West Germany.

Judy's Journey

Through the years, she worked at Evangeline Shoe in Manchester, Tel Labs and Computer Vision both formerly of Londonderry, Snow Nabstedt of Manchester. Most recently, she was a thirteen year employee of Wal-Mart Distribution Center in Raymond.

Judy enjoyed tending to her fish, gardening and caring for her collection of house plants and especially spending time with her grandchildren. She had been an avid candlepin bowler and in addition to many leagues, she had been a member of both the Professional Candlepin Bowling Association and the Senior Candlepin Bowling Association.

She leaves behind her husband of forty one years, Earle, and two grown children, Christina Thompson of Windham and Charles Whitcher of Deerfield, one sister, Helen of Lakeland, FL., two brothers, Michael of Fremont, Paul of Auburn and numerous aunts, uncles, cousins, nieces and nephews throughout the country.

In Her Life: She is survived by five grandchildren, Cynthia Fortier of Londonderry, Justin Broman and Andrew Whitcher of Deerfield, Samantha Thompson and Jeffrey Thompson, Jr. of Windham, and one great-granddaughter, Jaidyn Stultz of Londonderry.

Services: Calling hours will be on February 7, from 2 to 4 and 7 to 9 at Maiden-Petrin Funeral Home, Four Corners, Candia. A funeral service will take place on February 8, at 11 a.m. in the funeral home.

Graveside services will be held in the spring in Great Hill Cemetery in Chester, date to be announced.

Should anyone wish to make a donation in Judy's memory in lieu of flowers, please consider Breast Cancer or Brain Cancer focused charities.

Saturday, February 12, 2011

My intent today is to bring Judy's story to its conclusion and attempt to share her final farewell with those who were not able to join us this past week. It may take me a little longer than normal to compose the message—and myself—so please, bear with me.

During almost three weeks under the care of VNA Home Hospice, while steadily declining in strength and abilities, Judy passed from this life peacefully on February 4, 2011. She was where she wanted to be—at home and surrounded by family. The hospice staff was true to their word right up to and beyond the end. They calmly went into action and began to move us through the process of closure with dignity and gentle efficiency.

At the beginning of this journey, we knew that Judy's quality of life could be enhanced and prolonged, but that death would eventually result, if not from the disease itself, then likely from complications of it. By this time, I had set up the preliminary groundwork at the funeral home. The obituary still needed to be revised and made print-ready. We were also waiting to hear from Judy's sister and the other out-of-state folks as to their expected arrival so we could finalize the dates and times for the calling hours and memorial services.

I know the analogy may on the surface seem a poor choice, but the truth is, I felt as I could only imagine a nervous bride must feel just before the wedding day. I was worrying about every little detail and had convinced myself that the entire affair was going to be a complete disaster. As is most often the case, all of the details fell into place. To the outside world, everything appeared to go without a hitch. Isn't that the goal at these times?

All of the out-of-state folks arrived: Judy's sister and clan from Florida; my brother from Texas; and close friends from New Jersey, New York, Illinois, and Wisconsin. I was pleasantly surprised to see all of the friends who made the effort to travel such distances to be here for the services. I am only sorry that time was so short and the pressing events of the day were so concentrated that I was not able to spend more time with everyone.

I should note that all of the arrangements were Judy's own. She had spelled out in detail how she wanted things done. All I had to do was follow her directions (much like I had for the last 42 years). The calling hours were traditional: 2:00-4:00 p.m. and 7:00-9:00 p.m. on Monday, the 7th of February.

The afternoon hours were well attended. Although no official count was made, I think 50-60 people came by to pay their respects and offer condolences. All went as well as can be expected under such circumstances.

The evening hours were overwhelming. While again, no count was made, estimates were over 200 caring well-wishers. The procession never slowed for almost two hours. We were told that the line outside extended down the road and past the parking lot. The funeral director said that she had never hosted calling hours and a service so well attended. It was comforting to realize how many peoples' lives Judy had touched and to see the countless friends who took the time to express condolences to the family and say a final "Good-bye" to Judy. We were all amazed by the turnout.

Memorial services were set for Tuesday, February 8th. Rev. H. officiated over the proceedings.

Pastor H. had agreed to preside over the services; he was a longtime acquaintance of Judy's. As he revealed—much to the delight of the entire attending audience—at one time he was, as the term goes "sweet on her." They dated a few times a long time ago. I've always known this and never let an opportunity pass to lovingly chide Judy about going to see her "old boyfriend." The disclosure set the mood of the memorial service and placed an overflowing crowd at ease. I would estimate the number of attendees at about one hundred. We filled the main room and had seats set up in the outer hall and anteroom as well. Pastor H. delivered the eulogy, celebrating Judy's life in a beautiful service during which he shared her obituary and then tied Judy's natural life and the Lord's message of salvation and hope together. I think all in attendance were touched by his presentation. I heard nothing but high praise for the service. In addition to the formalities, several people spoke about Judy's impact on their lives. Their spontaneity added a personal touch which rounded out the event.

After the conclusion of the services at the funeral home, about 70 people joined us at a local eatery just two exits away. We spent the rest of the afternoon enjoying the establishment's excellent fare and socializing. We were joined by family, old friends, new friends, and all manner of folks to remember Judy and all she meant to so many. It was a joyful celebration. I am so glad that everyone there was able to join us in our time of reminiscing.

I feel I should assure everyone that in the time since Judy's passing and the celebration of her life, I am fine. Let me repeat that, because not everyone hears it the first time around. I am fine—and I will be fine.

Because we knew what the not-so-distant future ultimately held, Judy and I had much time to discuss what this phase of life might have in store for me. I do not have to second-guess what she wanted me to do. I am certain there will difficult times ahead, but I will face them and move on exactly as she wanted me to. I will never forget our time together and I will always cherish her memory, but I know that she did not want me to become a helpless shell of a man. I will honor her by doing as she wished and by getting on with whatever life may bring. Admittedly, I will have to learn how to be a bachelor for the first time in my life, but I have family and friends close by to lean on when needed. I also have a daughter who has recently taken on the role of housemother and does a nightly bed check to see if I am where I belong.

The final chapter for Judy will be written in the spring when the ground has finally thawed and dried out. Spring in New England also includes a pronounced Mud Season. Not much happens until that has concluded. The graveside services will be held after the earth returns to its ability to support both equipment and people. I will notify everyone, with as much lead time as I am provided from the funeral home, when that time comes.

Thank you one and all for your generous and endless support, prayers, and now condolences. You have all been a bigger part of this odyssey than you can imagine. Your expressions of faith and support have helped us immeasurably through what would have otherwise been some unbearable times. I sincerely mean it when I say, Thank You each and every one of you.

Earle

Given the fact that we live in New England and at the time of Judy's passing, the small town cemeteries generally do not conduct committal services when the ground is frozen, we had to wait for spring and all its glory to have the final services. At the memorial services in February, I was told to expect minimum lead time as to when the graveside ceremony would be held. As it turned out, I was given sufficient advance notice to advise everyone of the details. This allowed adequate time for all those who wanted to attend to make their arrangements.

May 6th again recurs in *Judy's Journey* one final time. It is the anniversary of the date of the very first communication to our friends and family in 2008; it marked the date when her first radiation treatment was scheduled in 2009; in 2010, Judy was recovering from an emotionally-shattering event and preparing for brain surgery on the following day.

It seemed strangely fitting that May 6th would also be the date for our final farewell at the gravesite. Now, May 6th brings with it closure for all of those who knew and loved Judy.

(It is also interesting to note that I had been given an additional date choice for the interment: that of Friday, May 13th. Two years prior, on Friday March 13, 2009, I made a determined decision not to send out an update until the following day. At the time, I indicated "though I was not particularly superstitious...why chance it?" I would not choose Friday, May 13th for Judy's final farewell for the same reason.)

Wednesday, April 13, 2011

I am at the same time both surprised and thrilled to be able to make this announcement with so much lead time. I have been in contact with the funeral director and the cemetery trustee and we have set a date for Judy's graveside services. While I realize that it will not be possible for all who might wish to do so to attend, I felt it only right to notify everyone who had been such an essential part of Judy's life and had played such an integral role in her struggle these last few years.

The services will be held at Great Hill Cemetery in Chester, NH, on May 6, 2011 at 1:00 p.m. Barring any unforeseen circumstances, we will be adhering to this schedule, rain or shine. Let us all hope for a beautiful, sunny, spring day to say our final farewell to Judy. Should anyone planning to attend need directions to the cemetery, feel free to contact me.

As I have done throughout Judy's tumultuous journey, I would like to take this opportunity to thank each of you for all your support, prayers, and heartfelt wishes. It is not possible to overstate how much that meant to both of us during those overwhelming days, as the disease forged mercilessly on despite our best efforts to halt its frightening course. We drew strength and courage from the knowledge that so many people were behind us and supporting us. Thank you all for that generous and unselfish support.

Earle

Friday, May 6, 2011

On Friday, May 6th, we gathered at Great Hill Cemetery in Chester to say our final "Goodbye" to Judy. To everyone who was able to join us, thank you for taking time out of your lives and schedules to do so. For the many friends and supporters who were such a big part of Judy's struggles and were not able to attend, I will try to describe how the day unfolded.

About a week prior to the scheduled graveside service, I started checking the long-range forecasts; it wasn't looking good. The prediction was for cloudy skies, showers, and rain. I'm still not entirely sure about the difference between showers and rain, but there it is.

Our only hope was the fact that the long-range projections around here are notoriously inaccurate.

As the day dawned, it was an absolutely beautiful, New England spring day. The temperature was in the low 70s and a slight breeze prevailed. The truth is, a little brisker breeze would have been welcome if it could have held the black fly population at bay. My best estimate put the gathering at sixty-plus attendees at the graveside services. Of those, about fifty or so were able to join us for a luncheon and to share a time of fellowship and reminiscing afterward.

Pastor H., the same minister who delivered such a beautiful eulogy at the memorial services, officiated at the graveside ceremony. Once again, he gave a masterful presentation. Many folks have commented to me about what a beautiful job he does ministering to people. We are grateful to have been able to avail ourselves of his services.

In the bright, spring sunshine, the white casket which I had chosen seemed to gleam. It was a striking sight; the faux-copper, exterior hardware affixed to the dazzling, white coffin, set against the green lawns. It was a fitting tribute for Judy.

As I mentioned, about fifty people joined us at a local restaurant for lunch and an opportunity to socialize following the graveside farewell. We had a great time getting together to remember Judy and all that she had meant to us. The gathering lasted a couple of hours and I think everyone enjoyed themselves.

The final step in the process will be the setting of the cemetery monument. Creating a fitting and lasting tribute to Judy, which would include reminders of those things she held dear in this life, is something that I put much thought into. It has been ordered. I have had one viewing of the proposed etchings and, after requesting a few changes, I am now waiting for the call to go in for the final approval. When the job is complete and the stone is set in place, I will send pictures to everyone so that you can all continue to be a part of our tribute to Judy.

As I have said so many times in the past, thank you all for your unwavering support, unconditional, heartfelt concern, and your prayers. It was the knowledge that so many folks were behind us during Judy's battle that made it possible for us to face those new challenges that never seemed to stop coming. Judy's fight is over now, but her memory and her legacy will live on in the hearts of all who knew and loved her. Thank you for being among those who have shared in the joy of having known her.

Thanks once again.

Earle

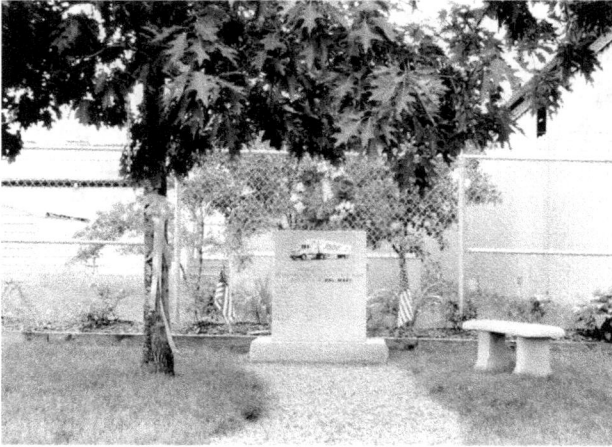

Memorial Garden at the Wal-Mart Distribution Center where Judy had worked

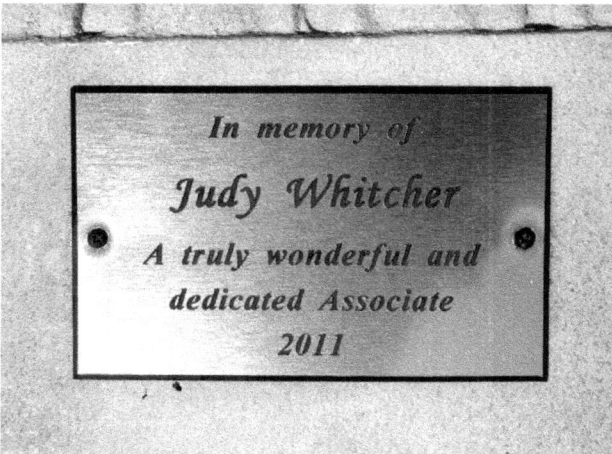

This plaque was affixed to the granite bench in Judy's memory
(seen to the right of monument in the picture above)

This concludes *Judy's Journey*. I hope that all who have joined us in sharing the story of Judy's courageous fight against the overwhelming odds that she faced can recognize the dignity and spirit that she displayed throughout the entire duration of her illness.

She taught us invaluable lessons during the course of her lifetime, but none were as poignant as those she taught us in her final years. Her energy and dynamic enjoyment of life, her tenacity and indomitable strength in the face of adversity, as well as her determination to press ever-forward in spite of life's challenges will forever be an inspiration to me and to all who have known her.

Though her time with us has ended, we all continue to celebrate her life and take joy in the fact that we were able to share the incredible journey that was her life. Judy's spirit will always live on in our hearts and memories

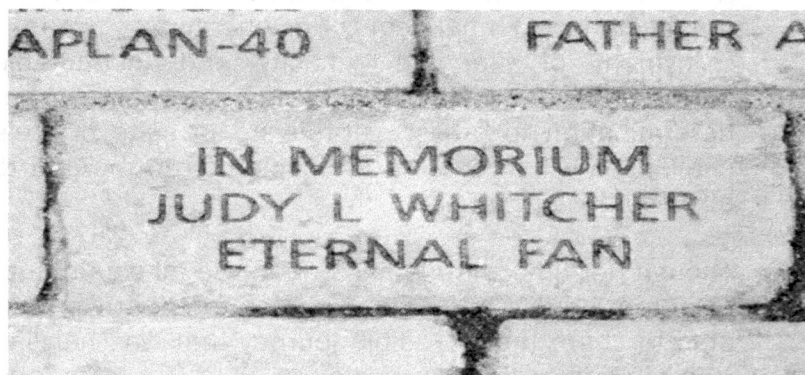

Judy's Memorial brick at Fenway Park in Boston, MA

Fenway Park is the home of the Boston Red Sox, one of Judy's favorite sports teams. This paving brick is located inside Gate C in the Pedro Martinez section.

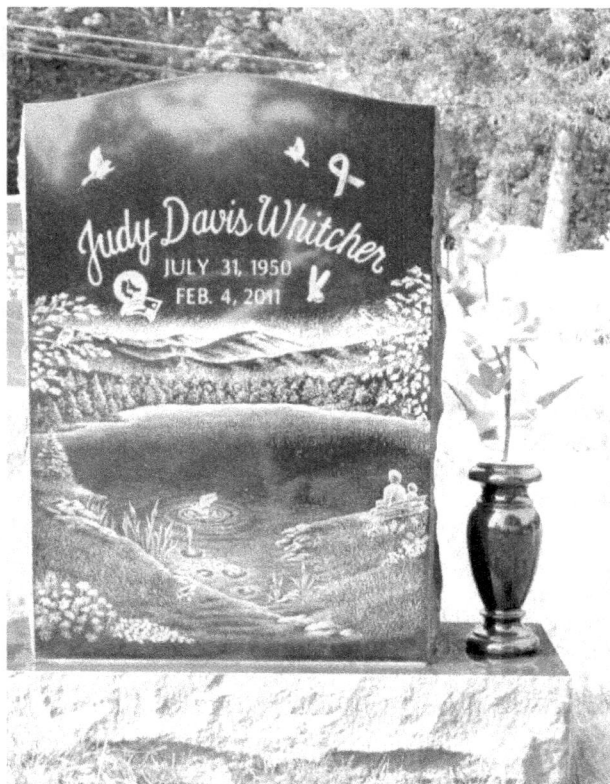

Judy's memorial monument: personalized with etchings of Judy sitting on a bench with a grandchild gazing at a country pond—complete with images of the flowers she nurtured and a little frog, such as the many she collected; in the upper right is a Breast Cancer ribbon representing her valiant fight; there are little birds like those she loved to feed; logos of her favorite sports teams: the Red Sox and the Patriots; as well as symbols of her pro-bowling career accomplishments. Discretely tucked away is the number 6830 denoting the Wal-Mart connection that had meant so much to Judy for many years.

Epilogue

Now that *Judy's Journey* has concluded I would like to take a moment or two for some final reflections.

The original intent of the updates that form the framework and comprise the majority of this volume was to relay up-to-date and accurate communications regarding Judy's condition, treatment, and progress as she battled the modern day demon known as Breast Cancer. At no time during the thirty-four months that these messages were being generated was anything remotely like the book that you have just read ever contemplated. The sole purpose of the updates was to spare family and friends the anguish of not knowing the truth and subsequently having to deal with the rumors that tend to fill the void when accurate information is absent.

Ironically, it was these same family and friends who urged me to follow through and develop what eventually became the tome you now hold in your hands. It will now forever be known as *Judy's Journey*. This effort has been a journey of sorts for me as well.

In the update of May 1, 2010, I mentioned how communicating through these updates had provided a dual benefit. Primarily, as intended, they served as a way for us to keep our family and friends informed of

Judy's progress without having to reiterate the painful details again and again. In retrospect, I cannot imagine the toll—in both time and energy—that it would have taken to have made the countless phone calls required to update folks about what had been transpiring—and re-living each event repeatedly in the process. Using the technology available, I could share the information once—initially for about 30 friends and family members, and later for well over 125 interested followers. The updates also provided an expressive outlet for me, permitting me to unburden myself of the strain and the feelings of helplessness which had so often intruded while we traveled that bumpy and convoluted road—the personal benefit was much like that derived from journaling. Though I didn't recognize it then, the messages also served to keep Judy in the thoughts and prayers of others on a consistent basis. Our contact group was "with us," supporting and encouraging us at every turn.

Was creating these messages a lot of work? Did they require a constant effort and significant emotional energy? Yes, to both questions, but we received so much more in return. If you, or a family member, are ever placed in this type of situation, consider communications such as these as an investment—one that will bless you many times over in return.

It should be noted that this book is far removed from anything that I have ever attempted before; but as it progressed and developed, it too became an outlet for my personal emotions. It truly became a cathartic exercise—a vehicle of healing—that has aided me through my own grieving process.

As I worked my way back over the many months of highs and lows that are a part of an experience such as this, I came to better understand and appreciate the courage and dignity that Judy displayed throughout the ordeal which was to punctuate her final three years in this, her earthly passage. It is not the inevitable final farewell that life holds in store for all of us; but rather the zest for life, which Judy held so dear, that I hope to have adequately conveyed to any who have chosen to partake of my meager literary efforts. Throughout her life, Judy modeled precious lessons for all of us pertaining to our daily lives. Her example remains valid, whether one is involved in a lethal struggle with some life-threatening disease or with the seemingly-mundane efforts required to sustain us through the challenges of our existence in an imperfect world.

You may recall in the opening paragraph of *Judy's Journey*, I stated that Judy's story was not about how the battle would culminate. The ultimate purpose was rather to chronicle her example as it unfolded, while she lived it before us, in the intervening period during the final years of her life.

We knew from the outset that unless God undertook to perform a miracle of total healing in her body, Judy would eventually succumb to the cancer, its complications, or to a metastasis of rogue cells which could affect her brain or other vital organs. Knowing this, we accepted every extension with which modern medical warfare could defer the naturally inevitable outcome, while praying and hoping that God's gracious mercy would give us more time together.

With every bit of optimism we could muster, we forged our way through the heights and the valleys ahead. We did everything in our power to help Judy achieve the priorities and objectives which were important to her. During the early days of her battle, we created a pictorial legacy accompanied by musical favorites. It was made possible by assembling hundreds of photos of family members—past and present—producing a Davis Family DVD. Judy shared the fruits of that endeavor with many of our extended family. Several people have commented on how much they treasure the preserved heritage, which would endure long after Judy's journey ended.

We traveled to our reunion in Alabama to share time with the families who had served with us in Germany. The one exception was that we never did make it to North Carolina—I guess, for whatever reason, that trip just wasn't meant to be. And finally, as an unexpected bonus, Judy would enjoy a few months of getting acquainted with her first great-grandchild. Jaidyn continues to thrill and amaze us all. She radiates that familiar zest for life that Judy so enthusiastically exhibited.

Judy came from humble beginnings. Though she may have lacked a college education, she possessed an understanding of the human condition, one that many never seem to grasp. She was caring and compassionate to those around her. Her friends, family, and co-workers all benefited from knowing her. She treated everyone with respect and, while she expected the same in return, she had the capacity to forgive when that was not the case.

As her husband of nearly 42 years, I knew her well. I knew who she was in public and I knew who she was in private when no one else was looking or judging her motives. Though not perfect by any stretch of the imagination, her life was a model that many people would do well to emulate. She was also a beacon of light, illuminating and demonstrating the way to face difficult situations with dignity, strength of character, determination, perseverance, and finally acceptance of her impending fate, as part of the will of God in her life. Most of us, myself included, can only hope to find that distinctive fortitude should we need it.

I consider myself privileged to have known Judy and to have shared a lifetime with her. It was my honor to have been by her side during those last months—an honor which I can only hope that I fulfilled in a worthy manner. I will be forever in her debt for the many ways in which she has enriched my life and I will always cherish and respect her memory.

During the time period that this manuscript was in the process of becoming what you now share, a much-admired vocalist released a new CD entitled "*Eleven.*" Martina McBride, an artist whom Judy and I both enjoyed, performs an emotionally-stirring rendition of one of the songs on that album that particularly resonated with me. Several close family members brought it to my attention as well, commenting upon the striking similarity to the journey that we had just completed. That song was entitled "*I'm Gonna Love You Through It*" (Lyrics by Ben Hayslip, Sonya Isaacs, and Jimmy Leary, 2011 WB Music Corp., Nashvistaville Songs; Sonya Isaacs Music; Universal Republic Records, a Division of UMG Recordings, Inc., 1755 Broadway, New York, NY). Having just accompanied me on *Judy's Journey*, if you have heard this song, you will know exactly what I mean. If you haven't, seek it out, and then sit quietly, and listen—really listen—to the words. Hear the story as it is revealed and you will understand why it struck such a chord with me: *"I know that you're afraid and I am too, but you'll never be alone, I promise you..."* These thoughts were constantly in my heart and mind; I could easily have spoken them to Judy so many times as we actually lived through the struggles. Besides being a beautiful song, it recounts an equally beautiful story of promise, faithfulness, and commitment. Ms. McBride reflects in her liner notes *"When I sang it I got chills from head to toe for the entire song. I still do when I sing it live. That has never happened to me before..."* The release of this CD occurred about six months after we said our final farewell to Judy. Because its theme so closely parallels my own recent journey, I have adopted it as my personal favorite and play it whenever I need a little help to get through my day. If the truth were told, it is playing as I write these very words.

Sometimes when it is quiet, I imagine I hear a voice announcing that "the ride is over; please remain seated until the roller coaster comes to a complete stop." I know Judy's ride isn't over, just changed—for the better I hope. I don't know what my next "ride" will be, but I know Judy would want me to follow her example, reach out for whatever life may have in store for me, and take the ride. I intend to honor that wish.

E. Whitcher

Reflections

Today is the day that my editor and I had set aside for what we hope to be the final edit prior to sending our project to the publisher. Today is the day that we should be putting our collective pens down for the last time; still, one more thought is coursing through my head and I am compelled to take this opportunity to share it.

I truly believe that each of us is put into our earthly existence for a reason. We may not always know what that reason is, and if we do, we may not always like it. Regardless of our circumstances; the reason endures. Our reason for being may have a profound effect on others throughout our entire lives. Remember the impact of George Bailey's life upon everyone that his touched in "It's a Wonderful Life."

During my lifetime, I have experienced—what I now recognize through the benefit of hindsight as—many close calls. There were times when, had the unfolding events been altered, even slightly, I might very well not have survived to tell this story today. I am recalling just a few.

There was the occasion when, at fourteen years of age, I was afflicted with a mysterious neurological ailment that had left me paralyzed from the waist down. Had it not

313

been for the unexpected visit of a concerned doctor to our home and an immediate transfer by ambulance to the hospital, I could have easily succumbed. I spent six weeks in the hospital before conditions began to improve and I was finally on the road to recovery.

Then there was the incident when a ladder went out from under me while I was thirty feet off the ground pulling cable in a machine shop. I fell between the heavy work benches to what could have been a messy demise. Spared, I came away with only bruises and a broken wrist. I also have vivid memories of the time that I failed to take the keys from a friend when he had no business being behind the wheel. While on the way to the store, we came so close to an oncoming vehicle that we struck each other's outside mirrors.

The difference between life and death is sometimes measured by minutes or inches. If I were to dwell on the subject, I could probably come up with more of these instances, but this should make my point. We are all here for a reason. At the time of these events, I had not yet fulfilled my purpose—thus I was spared.

I never considered myself to be a lucky person, so when these events occurred, I chalked them up to what little luck I had. Now, I believe that I was saved from harm's way because I had not yet fulfilled my life's intended purposes. During Judy's illness, I concluded that I was destined to be there for her in her time of need: to stand beside her, to support her, and to provide care and comfort to her. That seemed to appropriately fit the parameters of my circumstances at the time.

Today, I wonder if there wasn't an additional foreordained reason to my having shared so intimately in Judy's struggle. I wonder if this volume might be another element of my intended purpose in this life. What if all of the conditions that brought this story to light were set in place so that somewhere, at some moment in time, someone, who may be in need of assurance or encouragement, was to read about our challenges and discover a life-changing, possibly life-saving, glimmer of hope needed to surmount a seemingly-insurmountable dilemma? What if just one person was helped? What if *you* are intended to be that one person?

Should this work benefit any one of my readers, then perhaps one more infinitesimal piece of the puzzle of my life will have fallen into place. Possibly another part of the question that I continually ask myself—why am I here—will have been answered.

In closing, I have one final story I'd like to share. It is something that I heard about Michelangelo, the renowned sculptor and painter. As I heard it told, Michelangelo was ever-critical of his work. When he would visit individuals who now possessed some of his masterpieces, he would sometimes take out a brush that he'd cleverly tucked in his clothes and touch up here or there, where something didn't quite appear perfect to his eye. I will confess to sharing his self-critical trait. There is just a little bit of the perfectionist in me as well.

But now, after filling in the gaps and after much deliberation, I will finally lay down my "brush" and say "it is finished."

I wish you Godspeed and God bless.

E. Whitcher

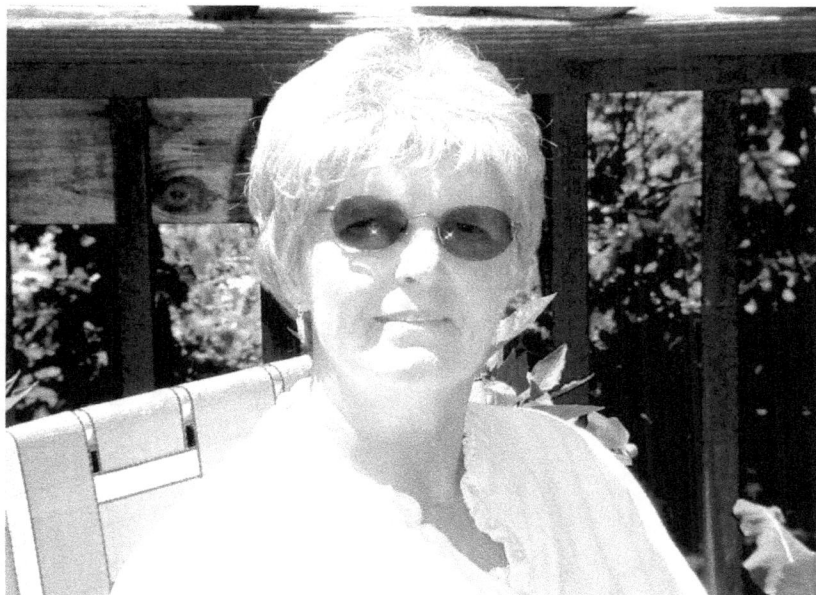

JUDY L. WHITCHER

1950 — 2011

E. Whitcher

ACKNOWLEDGEMENTS

My heartfelt thanks to all of the healthcare providers who worked so faithfully to meet Judy's needs throughout her illness: her PCP, Dr. T.; her neurosurgeon, Dr. J.; her radiologist, Dr. K.; her oncologist, Dr. B.; her general surgeon, Dr. H.; her GI surgeon, Dr. G.; her specialist and surgeon at the Breast Care Center, Dr. P.; her cardiologist, Dr. H.; her pulmonologist, Dr. F.; the nursing staff at the Elliot Hospital; the Hospice team at the Visiting Nurse Association; as well as local hospice volunteers.

I am deeply indebted to all of our—Judy's and my—friends and family members who supported us throughout the challenges that we faced with their kind thoughts, words of encouragement, and prayers. Many thanks for the cards, calls, flowers, and meals, as well as the rides to and from appointments when I could not be there. Thanks as well for the visits which continually reminded us that we were not alone.

I'd like to take this opportunity to express my appreciation to Rev. David Howe, Pastor of the United Pentecostal Church in Hudson, NH, for the spiritual support he provided during Judy's final days. In addition to that, his officiating at the memorial and committal services was second to none. For all of his efforts I will be eternally grateful.

Special acknowledgements to all of those "Update" recipients who valued these communications enough to have saved every one and then forwarded them back to me, thereby making this volume possible.

My heartfelt appreciation goes out to all of those who previewed the manuscript while it was in development. Cecile, Peggy, and Rebecca offered some insightful observations, suggestions, and resources that aided this endeavor.

My (sometimes grudging) thanks to A., Judy's and my cousin, who persistently urged me to author this work, contending that I "had already written the book" in the form of the updates. I finally relented and agreed to at least ask if anyone had saved them all—certain that <u>no one</u> would have and that I would be off the hook and could finally silence her. She was the driving force that made this rendering of *Judy's Journey* a reality. She insisted that someday I'd appreciate it, maybe...! ☺

Special thanks to Lynn Rockwell, Judy's and my neighbor, who so graciously agreed to review and edit the manuscript using her talents as a professional proofreader to offer her recommendations and comments. Her expertise served to further polish *Judy's Journey* and refine the final document as it was prepared for publication. (Lynn can be contacted at www.RedHotProofreading.com .)

Our sincere appreciation to RiverRun Select, RiverRun Bookstore, and Tom Holbrook. He worked patiently with my editor and me to modify our original manuscript into this volume. We both appreciated his willingness to share his professional expertise with the mechanics of the printing process without substantially altering the project we had brought to him.

And finally, I wish to acknowledge Anna Davis, my "chief editor" (and cheerleader) for the time and effort invested in editing, reviewing, and making suggestions regarding the manuscript. She also provided assistance detailing the medical aspects of treatment and terminology which contributed another perspective to this tribute to Judy.

As I put down my brush and close *Judy's Journey*, I would be remiss not to say a heartfelt thank you to my readers, one and all, for joining me on this journey.

E. Whitcher